DR ELISABETH KUBLE~ ~~~~
the author of the groundbrea
many other books which have ~~~
best-loved and most respected ...~ subject. She
                lives in Scottsdale, Arizona.

OTHER BOOKS BY ELISABETH KÜBLER-ROSS

Longing to Go Back Home (Germany)
Making the Most of the In-Between (Poland)
Unfolding the Wings of Love (Germany)
Death Is of Vital Importance
On Life After Death
AIDS: The Ultimate Challenge
On Children and Death
Remember the Secret
Working It Through
Living with Death and Dying
To Live Until We Say Goodbye
The Dougy Letter (Letter to a Dying Child)
Death: The Final Stage of Growth
Questions and Answers on Death and Dying
On Death and Dying

The WHEEL *of* LIFE

A Memoir of Living and Dying

ELISABETH KÜBLER-ROSS, M.D.

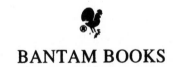

BANTAM BOOKS

LONDON · NEW YORK · TORONTO · SYDNEY · AUCKLAND

THE WHEEL OF LIFE
A BANTAM BOOK : 0 553 50544 0

Originally published in Great Britain by Bantam Press,
a division of Transworld Publishers

PRINTING HISTORY
Bantam Press edition published 1997
Bantam edition published 1998

7 9 10 8

Set in Garamond

Bantam Books are published by Transworld Publishers,
61–63 Uxbridge Road, London W5 5SA,
a division of The Random House Group Ltd,
in Australia by Random House Australia (Pty) Ltd,
20 Alfred Street, Milsons Point, Sydney, NSW 2061, Australia,
and in New Zealand by Random House New Zealand Ltd,
18 Poland Road, Glenfield, Auckland 10, New Zealand
and in South Africa by Random House (Pty) Ltd,
Endulini, 5a Jubilee Road, Parktown 2193, South Africa.

Printed and bound in Great Britain by
CPI Antony Rowe, Chippenham and Eastbourne

Papers used by Transworld Publishers are natural recyclable
products made from wood grown in sustainable forests.
The manufacturing processes conform to the environmental
regulations of the country of origin.

I dedicate this book to my children,
Kenneth and Barbara.

When we have done all the work we were sent to Earth to do, we are allowed to shed our body, which imprisons our soul like a cocoon encloses the future butterfly.

And when the time is right, we can let go of it and we will be free of pain, free of fears and worries—free as a very beautiful butterfly, returning home to God . . .

—from a letter to a child with cancer

Contents

❦

Acknowledgments

I want to use this opportunity to thank not just my good-weather friends but those who stuck with me in good times and bad.

David Richie, whom I met in the "old days" of Poland and Belgium and who despite his old age continues to keep contact and visit.

Ruth Oliver, whose love has always been unconditional.

Francis Luethy, who greatly helped me through my Virginia days.

I would also like to thank Gregg Furth, Rick Hurst, Rita Feild, Ira Sapin, Steven Levine and Gladys McGarrey for many, many years of friendship.

Cheryl, Paul and their son (my godchild) ET Joseph for their frequent visits.

Dr. and Dr. Durrer for their continued friendship.

Peggy and Alison Marengo for adopting seven AIDS babies and being an inspiration to us all. As well as my goddaughter Lucy.

And naturally my two sisters, Erika and Eva, as well as Eva's husband, Peter Bacher.

The WHEEL *of* LIFE

"THE MOUSE"
(early years)

The mouse enjoys getting in and out of everything, is lively and mischievous, is always ahead of the others.

"THE BEAR"
(early middle years)

The bear is very comfortable and loves to hibernate. It looks back at the early years and chuckles at the mouse as it runs around.

"THE BUFFALO"
(late middle years)

The buffalo loves to roam the prairies. It reviews life in a comfortable setting and is looking forward to lifting the heavy load and becoming an eagle.

"THE EAGLE"
(later years)

The eagle loves to soar high above the world, not to look down on people, but in order to encourage them to look up.

CHAPTER ONE

There Are No Accidents

❧

Maybe this will help. For years I have been stalked by a bad reputation. Actually I have been pursued by people who regard me as the Death and Dying Lady. They believe that having spent more than three decades in research on death and life after death qualifies me as an expert on the subject. I think they miss the point.

The only incontrovertible fact of my work is the importance of life.

I always say that death can be one of the greatest experiences ever. If you live each day of your life right, then you have nothing to fear.

Maybe this, what is certain to be my final book, will clear that up. It may also raise a few new questions and perhaps even provide the answers.

From where I sit today in the flower-filled living room of my home in Scottsdale, Arizona, the past seventy years of my life look extraordinary. As a little girl raised in Switzerland, I could never, not in my wildest dreams—and they were pretty wild—have predicted one day winding up as the world-famous author of *On Death and Dying*, a book whose exploration of life's final passage threw me into the center of a medical and theological controversy. Nor could I have imagined that afterward I would spend the rest of my life explaining that death does not exist.

According to my parents, I was supposed to have been a nice, churchgoing Swiss housewife. Instead I ended up an opinionated

15

psychiatrist, author and lecturer in the American Southwest, w[h]
communicates with spirits from a world that I believe is far mo[r]
loving and glorious than our own. I think modern medicine has
become like a prophet offering a life free of pain. It is nonsense.
The only thing I know that truly heals people is unconditional
love.

Some of my views are unconventional. For instance, throughout the past few years I suffered a half dozen strokes, including a
minor one right after Christmas 1996. My doctors warned, and
then begged me to give up smoking, coffee and chocolates. But I
still indulge in these tiny pleasures. Why not? It is my life.

That is how I have always lived. If I am opinionated and independent, if I am stuck in my ways, if I am a little off-center, so
what? That is me.

By themselves, the pieces do not seem to fit together.

But my experiences have taught me that there are no accidents
in life.

The things that happened to me *had* to happen.

I was destined to work with dying patients. I had no choice
when I encountered my first AIDS patient. I felt called to travel
some 250,000 miles each year to hold workshops that helped
people cope with the most painful aspects of life, death and the
transition between the two. Later in my life, I was compelled to
buy a 300-acre farm in rural Virginia, where I created my own
healing center and made plans to adopt AIDS-infected babies,
and, though it is still painful to admit, I see that I was destined
to be driven out of that idyllic place.

After announcing my intention of adopting AIDS-infected
babies in 1985, I became the most despised person in the whole
Shenandoah Valley, and even though I soon abandoned my
plans, there was a group of men who did everything in their
power short of killing me to get me to leave. They fired bullets
through my windows and shot at my animals. They sent the kind
of messages that made life in that gorgeous spot unpleasant and
dangerous. But that was my home and I stubbornly refused to
pack up.

I had moved to the farm in Head Waters, Virginia, ten years
earlier. The farm embodied all my dreams and I poured all the
money I earned from publishing and lectures into making it a

16

reality. I built my house, a neighboring cabin and a farmhouse. I constructed a healing center where I held workshops, allowing me to cut down on my hectic travel schedule. I was planning to adopt AIDS-infected babies, who would enjoy however many days remained of their lives in the splendor of the outdoors.

The simple life on the farm was everything to me. Nothing was more relaxing after a long plane flight than to reach the winding driveway that led up to my house. The quiet of the night was more soothing than a sleeping pill. In the morning, I awoke to a symphony of talking cows, horses, chickens, pigs, donkeys, llamas . . . the whole noisy menagerie, welcoming me home. The fields rolled out as far as I could see, glistening with fresh dew. Ancient trees offered their silent wisdom.

There was real work to be done. My hands got dirty. They touched the earth, the water, the sun. They worked with the material of life.

My life.

My soul was there.

Then, on October 6, 1994, my house was set on fire.

It burned down to the ground and was a total loss. All my papers were destroyed. Everything I owned turned to ash.

I was hurrying through the airport in Baltimore, trying to catch a plane home, when I got the news that it was ablaze. The friend who told me begged me not to go home, not yet. But my whole life I had been told not to become a doctor, not to talk with dying patients, not to start an AIDS hospice in prison, and each time I had stubbornly done what felt right rather than what was expected. This time was no different.

Everyone goes through hardship in life. The more you go through, the more you learn and grow.

The plane flight zoomed by. Soon I was in the backseat of a friend's car, speeding along the dark country roads. It was nearly midnight. From a distance of a few miles away, I spotted the first signs of smoke and flames. They stood out against a perfectly black sky. I could tell it was a big fire. Close up, the house, or what remained of it, was barely visible through the flames. I compared the scene to standing in the midst of hell. The firemen said they had never seen anything like it. The intense heat kept them at bay all night and through the morning.

17

Sometime late that first night I sought shelter in the nearby farmhouse, which had facilities for guests. I made myself a cup of coffee, lit a cigarette and considered the tremendous personal loss inside the raging furnace that was once my home. It was devastating, staggering, beyond comprehension. The list included diaries my father had kept of my childhood, my personal papers and journals, some 20,000 case histories pertaining to my research into life after death, my collection of Native American art, photos and clothing . . . everything.

For twenty-four hours I was in shock. I did not know how to react, whether to cry, scream, shake my fists at God or just gawk at the iron-fisted intrusion of fate.

Adversity only makes you stronger.

People always ask me what death is like. I tell them it is glorious. It is the easiest thing they will ever do.

Life is hard. Life is a struggle.

Life is like going to school. You are given many lessons. The more you learn, the harder the lessons get.

This was one of those times, one of those lessons. Since there was no use denying the loss, I accepted it. What else could I do? Anyway, it was just a bunch of stuff, and no matter how important or sentimental the meaning, nothing compared with the value of life. I was unharmed. My two grown children, Kenneth and Barbara, were alive. Some jerks might have succeeded in burning down my house and everything inside, but they were not able to destroy me.

When you learn your lessons, the pain goes away.

This life of mine, which began halfway around the world, has been many things—but never easy. That is a fact, not a complaint. I have learned there is no joy without hardship. There is no pleasure without pain. Would we know the comfort of peace without the distress of war? If not for AIDS, would we notice our humanity is in jeopardy? If not for death, would we appreciate life? If not for hate, would we know the ultimate goal is love?

As I am fond of saying: "Should you shield the canyons from the windstorms, you would never see the beauty of their carvings."

I admit that October night three years ago was one of those times when the beauty was hard to find. But during the course of my life, I had stood at similiar crossroads, searching the horizon for something nearly impossible to see. At those moments you can either hold on to negativity and look for blame, or you can choose to heal and keep on loving. Since I believe our only purpose for existing is to grow, I had no problem making a choice.

So a few days after the fire, I drove in to town, bought a change of clothes and got set for whatever was going to happen next.

In a way, that is the story of my life.

PART I

"THE MOUSE"

CHAPTER TWO

The Cocoon

Throughout life, we get clues that remind us of the direction we are supposed to be headed in. If you do not pay attention, then you make lousy choices and end up with a miserable life. If you stay focused, then you learn your lessons and have a full and good life, including a good death.

The greatest gift God has granted us is free will. It places responsibility for making the highest possible choices on our shoulders.

The first big decision I made solely by myself took place when I was in the sixth grade. Near the end of the semester, the teacher gave the class an assignment. We had to write an essay describing what we wanted to be when we grew up. In Switzerland, this particular task was a big event. It helped determine your future education. Either you received training in a profession or you went on to years of rigorous academic study.

I grabbed pencil and paper with unusual enthusiasm. But as much as I believed that I was charting my destiny, reality was different. Not all was left up to the child.

I only had to think back to the previous night. At dinner, my father had pushed his dishes aside and studied the faces of his family before making an important pronouncement. Ernst Kübler was a strong, tough man, with opinions to match. He was very strict and demanding with my older brother Ernst Junior and pushed him down a rigorous academic path. Now he was ready to reveal the future of his triplet daughters.

I was swept up by the drama as he told Erika, the frailest of the three girls, that she would follow an academic course. Then he told Eva, the least motivated, that she would receive a general education at a finishing school for girls. Finally his eyes turned to me and I prayed that he would grant my dream of becoming a physician.

Surely, he knew.

But the next moment I shall never forget.

"Elisabeth, you will work in my office," he said. "I need an efficient and intelligent secretary. That will be the place for you."

My heart sank. While I was growing up as a triplet, one of three identical girls, my whole life had been a struggle for my own identity. Now, once again, I was being denied the thoughts and feelings that made me unique. I imagined myself working in his office. I would have a clerical job. Sit at a desk all day. Write down numbers. The days would be as rigid as the lines on graph paper.

It was not me. From early on, I had an intense curiosity about life. I looked at the world with awe and reverence. I dreamed of becoming a country doctor, or better, practicing medicine among the poor in India the way my hero Albert Schweitzer did in Africa. I did not know where these ideas came from, but I did know that I was not cut out to work in my father's office.

"No, thank you!" I snapped.

In those days, such outbursts from children were not appreciated, especially in my household. My father turned red with anger. His temporal veins swelled with blood. Then he erupted. "If you don't want to work in my office, then you can spend the rest of your life as a maid," he yelled, and then stormed into his study.

"That's all right with me," I responded snappishly, and I meant it. I would rather work as a maid and hold fast to my independence than let someone, even my father, sentence me to life as a bookkeeper or secretary. For me, that would have been like going to prison.

All of that caused my heart to pound and my pen to fly the next morning in school when it came time to write our essays. Mine did not include a single mention of office work. Instead I wrote passionately about following Schweitzer into the jungle and researching life's many and varied forms. "I want to find out the purpose of life." Defying my father, I also stated that my dream included becoming a doctor. I did not care if he read my paper and got mad all over again. No one could take away my dreams. "One day I bet I can do it on my own feet," I said. "We should always reach for the highest star."

*   *   *

The questions of my childhood: Why was I born a triplet with no clear identity of my own? Why was my father so tough? Why was my mother so loving?

They had to be. That was part of the plan.

I believe every person has a guardian spirit or angel. They assist us in the transition between life and death and they also help us pick our parents before we are born.

My parents were a typical upper-middle-class, conservative couple in Zurich, Switzerland. Their personalities proved the old axiom that opposites attract. My father, the assistant director of the city's biggest office supply company, was a well-built, serious, responsible and thrifty man. He had dark brown eyes that saw only two possibilities in life—his way and the wrong way.

But he also had a terrific enthusiasm for life. He led loud sing-alongs around the family piano and he lived to explore the wondrous beauty of the Swiss landscape. A member of the prestigious Zurich Ski Club, my father was happiest when hiking, climbing or skiing in the mountains. It was a love he passed on to his children.

My mother had a fit, suntanned and healthy look even though she did not participate in outdoor activities with the same zeal as my father. Petite and attractive, she was a practical homemaker, and proud of her skills. She was a fine cook. She sewed many of her own clothes, knitted warm sweaters, kept a neat home and tended a garden that drew many admirers. She was a fine asset to my father's business. After my brother was born, she dedicated herself to being a good mother.

But she wanted a pretty little daughter to complete the picture. She got pregnant for a second time without any difficulty. As she went into labor on July 8, 1926, she prayed for a curly-haired muffin she could dress in fancy doll-like clothes. Dr. B., an elderly obstetrician, helped her through the pains and contractions. My father, notified at work of my mother's condition, arrived at the hospital at the culmination of nine months of anticipation. The doctor reached down and caught a baby, the smallest newborn anyone in the delivery room had ever seen born alive.

That was my arrival. I weighed two pounds. The doctor was shocked by my size, or rather my lack of it. I looked like a little mouse. No one expected me to survive. However, as soon as my father heard my first cry, he dashed to the phone in the hallway outside and informed his mother, Frieda, that she had another grandson.

Once he ran back to the delivery room, he was corrected. "Frau Kübler," the nurse said, "actually gave birth to a daughter." My father was told that often such tiny babies cannot be correctly identified at birth. So he hurried back to the phone and told his mother that she had her first granddaughter.

"We plan to call her Elisabeth," he said proudly.

By the time my father reentered the delivery room to comfort my mother, he was in for another surprise. A second baby girl had also been born. Like me, she was a fragile two-pounder. After my father finished informing his mother of the additional good news, he found my mother still in considerable pain. She swore that she was not finished, that she was going to have another child. My father thought it was nonsense caused by fatigue, and the old experienced doctor reluctantly agreed.

But suddenly my mother began having more contractions. She started to push and moments later gave birth to a third daughter. This one was large, six and a half pounds, which was triple the weight of either of the other two. And this one had a full head of curls! My exhausted mother was thrilled. She finally had the little girl she had dreamed of for the past nine months.

Dr. B., an elderly woman, thought of herself as a clairvoyant. We were the first set of triplets she had ever delivered. She studied our faces in close detail and gave my mother predictions about each of us. She said that Eva, the last one born, would always remain "closest to her mother's heart," while Erika, the second child, would always "choose a path in the middle." Then Dr. B., gesturing at me, remarked how I had shown the others the way and added, "You will never have to worry about this one."

All the local papers carried the exciting news of the Kübler triplets in the next day's edition. Until she saw the headlines, my grandmother thought my father had been playing a stupid joke. The celebrating went on for days. Only my brother failed to share the excitement. His days as a charmed little prince ended abruptly. He found himself buried under an avalanche of diapers. Soon he would be pushing a heavy carriage up hills and watching his three sisters sit on identical potties. I am quite certain that the lack of attention he received explains his distance from the family later on.

For me, being a triplet was a nightmare. I would not wish it on my worst enemy. I had no identity apart from my sisters. We looked alike. We received the same presents. Teachers gave us the same grades. On walks in the park, passersby asked which one was which. Sometimes my mother admitted even she did not know.

It was a heavy psychological weight to carry around. Not only was I born a two-pound nothing and given a slim chance at survival; my whole childhood was spent attempting to figure out who I was. I always felt that I had to work ten times harder than everyone else and do ten times more to prove myself worthy . . . of something . . . worthy of living. It was a daily torture.

Only as an adult did I realize it had been a blessing instead. Those circumstances are what I had chosen for myself before entering the world. They may not have been pleasant. They may not have been what I wanted. But they were what gave me the grit, determination and stamina for all the work that lay ahead.

CHAPTER THREE

A Dying Angel

After four years of raising triplets in a cramped Zurich apartment, where we had no space or privacy, my parents rented a charming, three-story country home in Meilen, a traditional Swiss village on the lake a half-hour train ride from Zurich. It was painted green, which inspired us to call it "the Green House."

Our new home sat on a grassy hill overlooking the village. It had lots of Old World character and a tiny grass yard where we were able to run and play. There was a garden which supplied us with fresh vegetables from our own harvest. Energetic, I took to the outdoors, very much my father's child. I sometimes spent all day roaming the woods and meadows and chasing birds and animals.

I have two very early memories from this time, both very important in shaping the person I would become.

The first was my discovery of a picture book on life in an African village, which sparked my lifelong curiosity about the world's different cultures. I was immediately fascinated by the photos of the dark-skinned children. I tried understanding them better by inventing a make-believe world that I could explore, including a secret language that I shared only with my sisters. I pestered my parents for a black-faced doll, which was impossible to find in Switzerland. I even gave up playing with my doll collection till I had some with black faces.

When I heard about a new African exhibition opening at the zoo in Zurich, I sneaked off to see it for myself. I caught the train, as I had done previously with my parents, and easily found the zoo. I watched the African drummers create the most beautiful, exotic-sounding rhythms. Meanwhile, the entire town of Meilen was out searching for the naughty Kübler runaway. Little did I know the concern I had created when I wandered in that night, but I was properly punished.

Around the same time, I also remember attending a horse race with my father. Since I was so tiny, he pushed me to the front of the grown-ups in order to see better. I sat on the moist spring grass all afternoon. Despite a slight chill, I sat still in order to enjoy the closeness of these beautiful horses. I developed a cold soon afterward and the next thing I remember was a night sleep-walking in a delirious state throughout the basement of our house.

Totally disoriented when found by my mother, she took me into the guest bedroom where she could keep an eye on me. It was the first time I had ever slept away from my sisters. I had a high fever, which was rapidly turning into pleurisy and pneumonia. I knew my mother was upset with my father for being away on a ski trip and leaving her with her tiresome trio and little son.

At 4 A.M., with my fever spiking, my mother called one neighbor to watch my brother and sisters and then she asked another neighbor, Mr. H., who owned a car, to drive us to the hospital. She wrapped me in several blankets and held me in her arms while Mr. H. drove very fast to the children's hospital in Zurich.

This was my introduction to hospital medicine, and unfortunately it is memorable for being unpleasant. The examining room was cold. No one said a word to me. Not "Hello." Not "How are you?" Nothing. A doctor yanked the cozy blankets off my shivering body and quickly undressed me. He asked my mother to leave the room. Then I was weighed, poked, prodded, asked to cough and treated like a thing rather than a little girl as they sought the cause of my problems.

The next thing I remember is waking up in a strange room. It was actually more like a glass cage. Or a fishbowl. It was perfectly silent. An overhead light stayed on practically around the clock. For the next few weeks, I saw people in white lab coats come and go without uttering a single word or offering a friendly smile.

30

There was another bed in the fishbowl. It was occupied by a little girl who was two years older than I. She was very frail and her skin was so pale and sickly it appeared to be translucent. She reminded me of an angel without wings, a little porcelain angel. No one ever visited her.

She drifted in and out of consciousness, so we never actually spoke. But we were very comfortable with each other, relaxed and familiar. We stared into each other's eyes for immeasurable periods of time. It was our way of communicating. We had long, deep and meaningful conversations without ever making a single sound. It was a kind of simple transference of thoughts. All we had to do was open our young eyes to start the flow. Oh, my, there was so much to say.

Then one day, shortly before my own illness took a drastic turn, I opened my eyes from a dreamy sleep and saw my roommate looking at me, waiting. We then had a beautiful, very moving and purposeful discussion. My little porcelain friend told me that she would be leaving later that night. I grew concerned. "It's okay," she said. "There are angels waiting for me."

That evening she stirred more than normal. As I tried to get her attention, she kept looking past me, or through me. "It's important that you keep fighting," she explained. "You're going to make it. You're going to return home with your family." I was so happy, but then my mood changed abruptly. "What about you?" I asked.

She said that her real family was "on the other side" and assured me that there was no need to worry. We traded smiles before drifting back to sleep. I had no fear of the journey my new friend was embarking on. Nor did she. It seemed as natural as the sun going down every night and the moon taking its place.

The next morning I noticed that my friend's bed was empty. None of the doctors or nurses said a word about her departure, but I smiled inside, knowing that she had confided in me before leaving. Maybe I knew more than they did. Certainly I have never ever forgotten my little friend who appeared to die alone but was, I am sure, attended to by people on a different plane. I knew she had gone off to a better place.

As for me, I was not so certain. I hated my doctor. I blamed her for not allowing my parents to get any closer than the other side of the window. They stared at me from outside while I desperately needed a hug. I wanted to hear their voices. I wanted to feel the warm skin of my parents and to hear my siblings laugh. Instead my parents pressed their faces against the glass. They held up pictures my sisters sent; they smiled and waved; and that was the extent of their visits while I was in the hospital.

My only pleasure was peeling the dead skin off my blistered lips. It felt good, and it irritated the heck out of my doctor. She hit my hand constantly and threatened that if I did not stop she would tie my arms down and immobilize me. Defiant and bored, I continued. I could not stop myself. It was the only fun I had. But one day after my parents left, that cruel doctor came into my room, saw my lips bleeding and tied my arms down so that I could not touch my face anymore.

Instead I used my teeth. My lips bled constantly. The doctor hated me for being a stubborn, unruly, disobedient child. But I was none of that. I was sick and lonely and craving the warmth of human contact. I used to rub my feet and legs together to feel the comforting touch of human skin. This was no way to treat a sick child, and no doubt there were children much sicker than I who had it even worse.

Then one morning several doctors huddled around my bed, whispering something about my needing a blood transfusion. Early the next day my father walked into my desperately empty and desolate room, looking quite large and heroic. He announced that I was going to receive some of his own "good Gypsy blood." Suddenly the room brightened. We lay down on neighboring stretchers and tubes were stuck in our arms. The suction-circulating-pumping device was cranked by hand and looked like a coffee grinder. Father and I both stared at the crimson tubes. Each time the crank was turned, it pulled the blood from my father's tube and forced it into mine.

"This will get you over the brink," he said encouragingly. "Soon you will be able to go home."

Naturally I believed every word.

I was depressed when the procedure ended, because then my father got up and left me alone again. But after several days, my fever went down and my cough subsided. Then one morning my father showed up again. He ordered me to raise my spindly body out of bed and walk down the hallway into a little dressing room. "There is a little something waiting there for you," he said.

Though I was uncertain on my feet, my soaring spirit carried me down the hall, where I imagined my mother and sisters were prepared to surprise me. Instead I entered an empty room. The only thing in it was a small leather suitcase. My father stuck his head in and told me to open the case and quickly get dressed. I was weak and worried about falling, never mind that I barely had the strength to open the suitcase. But I did not want to disobey my father and perhaps miss a chance to go home with him.

So I used all my strength to open the suitcase. Then I found the best surprise of my life. Inside, my clothes were neatly folded, obviously my mother's work, and poised on top of everything was a black doll. It was the kind of black doll I had dreamed about for months. I picked it up and started to cry. I had never had a doll of my own before. Nothing. Not a toy or even an article of clothing that I did not share with my sisters. But this black doll was obviously mine, all mine, clearly distinguishable from Eva's and Erika's white dolls. I was so happy I felt like dancing—if only my weak legs would have allowed it.

At home, my father carried me upstairs and put me in bed. For the next few weeks, I ventured only as far as the comfortable chair on the balcony, where I rested with my prized black doll in my arms, letting the sun warm my skin as I gazed admiringly at the trees and flowers where my sisters played. I was so happy to be home I didn't mind that I could not play with them.

Sadly, I missed the start of school, but one sunny day my favorite teacher, Frau Burkli, showed up at our house with the whole class. They assembled below my balcony and serenaded me with my favorite happy songs. Before leaving, my teacher handed me an adorable black bear that was filled with the most delicious chocolate truffles, which I devoured at a record pace.

Slowly but surely, I returned to normal, and as I realized much later in my life, long after I had joined the ranks of those white-jacketed hospital doctors, it was due largely to the best medicine in the world: the care, comfort and love I got at home . . . and a few chocolates too!

CHAPTER FOUR

My Black Bunny

M y father delighted in taking snapshots of family occasions, which he meticulously arranged in photobooks. He also kept detailed diaries of who uttered the first words, learned to crawl, walk, said something funny or insightful—precious mementos that always caused me to smile until most of them were destroyed. Thankfully, they are all still lodged in my mind.

Christmas was the best time of year. In Switzerland, every child works hard to come up with handmade gifts for all the family members and close relatives. In the days preceding Christmas, we sat together knitting covers for clothes hangers, embroidering fancy hankies and thinking of new stitches for tablecloths and doilies. I was so proud of my brother when he brought home a shoe-shine kit he had made in his woodworking shop at school.

My mother was the best cook in the world, but she took great pride in making special and new menus over the holidays. She was very picky about where she bought her meat and vegetables, and she did not shy away from walking miles to get one special thing from a store clear across the village.

Although in our eyes my father was thrifty, he would always bring a bouquet of fresh anemones, ranunculus, daisies and mimosas home for Christmas. I can still smell the scent of those flowers every December by just closing my eyes. He also brought home cartons of dates, some dried figs and other treats that made the Advent season mystical and special. My mother would fill all the vases with flowers and fir branches and decorate the house especially nice. There was always an air of anticipation and excitement.

On December 25, my father took all of us children on a long walk in search of the Christ child. A good storyteller, he made us believe that the glitter in the snow was a sign that the Christ baby was just a few moments ahead of us. We never questioned him while hiking through forests and over hills, always hoping we would be able to see him with our own eyes. The hike lasted for several hours, until darkness, when my father, with a defeated sigh, decided it was time to return home so Mother would not worry.

But no sooner did we arrive at the garden than my mother, bundled up in a thick coat, returned home herself, apparently from some late shopping. We would all walk into the house simultaneously and with great excitement discover that the Christ child had apparently been in our living room and lit all the candles on a huge and exquisitely decorated Christmas tree. There were packages under the tree. We ate a big feast as the candles flickered.

Afterward, we retired to the drawing room, which doubled as the music room and library, and my family would start singing the old and beloved Christmas songs. My sister Eva played the piano and my brother accompanied on the accordion. My father had a gorgeous tenor singing voice, and everybody joined in. Then my father read a Christmas story with the kids sitting spellbound at his feet. While my mother relit the candles on the tree and prepared dessert, we snuck around the tree, trying to figure out the contents of each package. Finally, after dessert, we opened the packages and then played games until bedtime.

On normal working days, my father used to leave early in the morning to catch the train to Zurich. He returned for lunch and then left again for the train station afterward. That left my mother very little time to make the beds and clean the house before preparing lunch, which was usually four courses and the main meal of the day. We all had to be at the table, and we got "the eagle eye" from my strict disciplinarian father if we made too much noise or did not finish everything on our plates. He rarely had to raise his voice, so when he did everybody quickly behaved. If not, he invited

36

us into his study and we knew what that meant.

I cannot remember my father ever losing his temper with Eva or Erika. Erika was unusually good and quiet all of the time. Eva was my mother's favorite. So Ernst and I were the usual targets. My father had nicknames for all of us: Erika as *Augedaechli*, which meant the lid over the eyeball, a symbolic gesture of how close he felt to her, and perhaps because he always saw her half-dreaming, half-asleep with her eyes almost closed. Because I always hopped from branch to branch, he called me *Meisli*, or little sparrow, and changed that to *Museli*, or little mouse, because I never sat still. Eva was called *Leu*, which means Lion, probably because of the amount of gorgeous hair she had as well as her good appetite! Ernst was the only one called by his original name.

In the evening, long after we returned from school and my father from work, we all gathered in the music room and sang. My father, a much-in-demand entertainer at the prestigious Zurich Ski Club, made sure we learned hundreds of popular ballads and songs. Over time, it was obvious that Erika and I had no musical ability and added only off-key notes to an otherwise lively concert. As a result, my father delegated us to kitchen duty. Almost daily, while the others sang, Erika and I ended up washing the dinner dishes and singing by ourselves. But we did not mind. When we finished, rather than join the others, we sat on the counter, sang by ourselves and sent in requests for favorites like "Ave Maria," "*Das alte Lied*" and "Always." Those were the best times.

Come bedtime, we shared identical beds and linen and put our identical clothes on identical chairs for the next morning. From dolls to books, everything was the same for the three of us. It was maddening. I remember my poor brother being used as a watchdog during our potty sessions. His job was to make sure I did not spring up early and run away before my sisters were finished. I resented this procedure and felt like I had been put in a straightjacket. All of this fanned my desire for my own identity.

At school, I was much more of an individual than my sisters. An excellent student, especially in math and languages, but I was best known for defending weak, helpless or handicapped children from trouble-makers. My fists pummeled the backs of the school's bullies so often that my mother was accustomed to the butcher boy, the town gossip, passing by our house after class and saying, "Betli will be late today. She's beating up one of the boys." My parents never got mad, since they knew I only protected those who could not defend themselves.

Unlike my sisters, I was also very involved with pets. At the end of kindergarten a close family friend returned from Africa and gave me a little monkey I named Chicito. We quickly became special friends. I also collected all sorts of animals and ran a makeshift hospital in the basement for injured birds, frogs and snakes. Once I nurtured a hurt crow back to health so it was able to fly away again. I guessed that animals knew instinctively who to trust.

That was certainly true of the dozen or so bunnies we kept in a little coop out in the garden. I was primarily responsible for cleaning their house, making sure they were fed and playing with them. Even though my mother put rabbit stew on the menu every few months, I conveniently never thought of how the rabbits got in the stewpot. On the other hand I did notice the rabbits only approached the gate when I entered, never when anybody else from my family walked in. This favoritism inspired me to spoil them even more. At least they could distinguish me from my sisters.

After they started multiplying, my father decided to reduce their numbers and only keep a certain minimum of rabbits. I do not understand why he did this. They cost nothing to feed, since they ate dandelions and grass, and there was no shortage of either in our yard. But he must have figured that he was saving money somehow. One morning he asked my mother to make a rabbit roast. Then he got hold of me. "Take one of your rabbits to the butcher on your way to school," he said. "Then bring it back over the lunch break so Mother can cook it in time for dinner."

Though rendered speechless by the thought of what he requested, I obeyed. Later that night, I watched my family eat "my" bunny. I nearly choked when my father suggested I try a little bite. "Perhaps a leg," he said. I stubbornly refused and managed to avoid an "invitation" to my father's study.

This drama repeated itself for months, until the only rabbit left was Blackie, my favorite. He was a big, fat ball of fluff. I loved to cuddle him and unburden all my secrets. He was a great listener, a wonderful shrink. I was convinced he was the only living creature in the whole world who loved me unconditionally. Then came the day I dreaded. After breakfast, my father told me to take Blackie to the butcher. I walked outside shaking and distraught. As I scooped him up, I confessed what I'd been ordered to do. Blackie looked at me, his pink nose twitching.

"I can't do it," I said, and placed him on the ground. "Run away," I begged. "Go." But he did not budge.

Finally I ran out of time. School was about to start. So I grabbed Blackie and ran to the butcher shop, tears running down my cheeks. Poor Blackie sensed something dreadful was about to happen, I have to think. I mean, his heart was beating as fast as mine as I handed him to the butcher and hurried off to school without saying goodbye.

I spent the rest of the day thinking about Blackie. I wondered if he had been killed already, if he knew that I loved him and would miss him forever. I regretted not having said goodbye. All of these questions I asked myself, not to mention my attitude, planted the seeds for my future work. I hated the way I felt and blamed my father.

After school, I walked slowly into the village. The butcher was waiting in the shop's doorway. As he handed me the bag containing Blackie, he said, "It's a damn shame you had to bring this rabbit. In a day or two, she would have had bunnies." (I hadn't known that Blackie was a female.) I did not think I could feel any worse, but I did. I deposited the still-warm bag on the counter. Later I sat at the table and watched my family eat my bunny. I did not cry. I did not want my parents to know how much they had hurt me.

I reasoned that they obviously did not love me, and so I had to learn to be tough. Tougher than anyone.

As my father complimented my mother on the delicious meal, I told myself, "If you can make it through this, then you can make it through anything in life."

When I was ten my father moved us to a much larger house, one we referred to as "the Big House," farther up in the hills above the village. We had six bedrooms, but my parents still kept us three girls in the same room. By then, the only space that mattered to me was outdoors. We had a spectacular yard, two acres of lawn, flowers and a garden, clearly the source of my lifelong interest in growing anything that blooms. We were also surrounded by the picture-book-pretty farms and vineyards, and far in the background there were craggy snowcapped mountains.

I roamed all over the countryside, searching for wounded birds, cats, snakes, frogs and various other animals. I carried them back to our basement, where I set up a fine laboratory. I proudly referred to it as "my hospital." For my less fortunate patients, I created a cemetery under a willow tree and kept the shaded area decorated with flowers.

My parents did not shield me from life and death as it happened naturally, which allowed me to absorb the different circumstances as well as people's reactions. In third grade, my class was introduced to a new girl named Suzy. Her father, a young doctor, had just moved his family to Meilen. It was not easy starting a new medical practice in a small village, and the father had a hard time getting patients. But everyone thought Suzy and her younger sister were adorable.

Then a few months later Suzy stopped going to school. Soon word spread that she was seriously ill. Everyone in town blamed her father for not making her better. Therefore he must not be a good doctor, they reasoned. But not even the best physicians in the world could have helped. Suzy, it turned out, had contracted meningitis.

The whole town, including the schoolchildren, followed her gradual decline: first paralysis set in, then deafness, and finally she lost her eyesight. The villagers, though saddened for her family, were like most small-town people: they feared the horrible illness might find its way into their homes if they got too close. Consequently, the new family was practically shunned and left alone in a time of great emotional need.

It disturbs me to think about that now, even though I was among a group of Suzy's schoolmates who continued to have contact. I gave her sister notes, drawings and wildflowers to take home. "Tell Suzy that we are thinking of her," I said. "Tell her that I miss her."

I will never forget that when Suzy died her bedroom curtains were shut. I recall being sad that she was closed off from the sunshine, the birds, the trees and all the lovely sounds and sights of nature. It did not seem right to me. Nor did the outpouring of sadness and grief that followed, since I thought most Meilen residents felt relieved that the ordeal was finally over. With no reason to stay, Suzy's family moved away.

I was much more positively impressed by the death of one of my parents' friends. He was a farmer, probably in his fifties. Years earlier he had been the one who had rushed my mother and me to the hospital when I had pneumonia. His death came after he fell from an apple tree and broke his neck, but it did not kill him immediately.

At the hospital, doctors told him they were helpless, and so he insisted on being taken home to die. There was plenty of time for his family, relatives and friends to say goodbye. On the day we went, he was surrounded by his family and children. His room overflowed with wildflowers, and his bed was positioned so that he could look out the window on his fields and fruit trees, literally the fruits of his labor that would survive the drift of time. The dignity and love and peace I saw made a lasting impression.

The next day he died, and we returned that afternoon to view his body. I was a very reluctant participant, not eager at all for the experience of the lifeless body. Some twenty-four hours earlier this man, whose children attended school with me, had uttered my name, a painful but heartfelt "little Betli." But the viewing turned out to be a fascinating moment. Gazing at his body, I realized that he was no longer there. Whatever force and energy gave him life, whatever it was that we mourned, had vanished.

In my mind, I compared his death with Suzy's. Whatever happened to her unfolded in the dark, behind drawn curtains that prevented even the warm rays of sunshine from entering her final moments. The farmer had died what I now call a good death— at home, surrounded by love and given respect, dignity and affection. His family said all they had to say and grieved without any regrets or unfinished business.

From my few experiences, I realized that death was something that you could not always control. But given some choice, this felt right.

CHAPTER FIVE

Faith, Hope and Love

I was lucky in school. My interest in math, and academics in general made me one of those odd children who loved attending school. But I had the opposite reaction to my mandatory weekly religious studies. It was too bad, because as a child I definitely had a spiritual inclination. But Pastor R., the town's Protestant minister, taught the scripture on Sundays by emphasizing fear and guilt, and I did not identify with *his* God.

He was a cold, brutish, unsophisticated man. His five children, who knew how unchristian he truly was, showed up at school hungry and with black-and-blue marks covering their bodies. The poor things looked tired and worn out. We sneaked them sandwiches for belated breakfasts and shoved sweaters and pillows under their rear ends so they could tolerate sitting on wooden benches outside. Eventually their family secrets filtered into the schoolyard—each morning their most revered father smacked the heck out of them with whatever he found handy.

Instead of confronting him about his terribly abusive behavior, the adults admired his eloquent, highly dramatic sermons, but all of us kids who were subjected to his dictatorial manner of teaching and rigid discipline knew better. A sigh during his lecture, or a slight turn of the head, resulted in a sharp crack of a wooden ruler on your arm, head or ear, or worse.

He fell out of my favor, as did religion in general, the day my sister Eva was asked to recite a Psalm. We had memorized the Psalm the previous week. My sister knew it perfectly. But before she finished, the girl next to her coughed. Pastor R. mistakenly thought that she had whispered the Psalm into my sister's ear. Without asking any questions, he grabbed each of their braids and bashed their heads together. The crack of their bones produced a sound that made the entire class shudder.

That was too much, and I exploded. I threw the black psalm-book in my hand at his face. It hit him smack in the kisser. He was stunned and looked directly at me, but I was too incensed to be intimidated. I screamed that he was not practicing what he preached. "You are not an example of a caring, compassionate, loving and understanding minister," I shrieked. "I don't want to be a part of any religion you are teaching!" Then I dashed out of school and swore never to go back.

On my way home, I was upset and frightened. Even though I knew my action was justified, I feared the consequences. I imagined being expelled from school. But the bigger unknown was my father. I did not even want to think about how he would punish me. Then again, he was not a fan of Pastor R. The pastor had recently selected our neighbors as the most exemplary Christian family in the village, yet every night we heard the parents scream and fight and beat their children. On Sunday they put up a lovely front. But my father wondered how Pastor R. could be so blind.

On the way home, I stopped to rest in the shade offered by one of the large trees on the outskirts of a vineyard. This was my church. The open fields. The trees. Birds. Sunshine. I had no doubt about the sanctity and awe inspired by Mother Nature. Timeless and trustworthy in her appearance. Beautiful and most beneficent in her treatment of others. Forgiving. This was my refuge from trouble, my safe haven from phony grown-ups. This truly bore the hand of God.

My father would understand. He was the one who taught me to worship nature's generous splendor by taking us on long hikes in the mountains, where we would investigate the moors and meadows, swim in clear, crisp brooks and cut our own paths through thick forests. He took us on pleasant spring hikes and also dangerous expeditions through the snow. We caught his enthusiasm for the tallest mountains, a half-hidden edelweiss in a rock or the glimpse of a rare alpine flower. We savored the beauty of a sunset. We also respected the danger, such as the time when I took a near-fatal fall into a deep glacial crevice—and was only able to be rescued because I was wearing my safety rope.

Those tracks we laid were imprinted on our souls forever.

Before going home, where by now news of my run-in with Pastor R. was certain to have reached, I crawled into a secret spot within the meadow behind our house. I considered it to be the holiest spot in the entire world. Located in the center of a piece of virgin wilderness so thick with growth that no human being had penetrated it—except for me—was an enormous rock, perhaps five feet high and covered with moss, lichen, salamanders and creepy crawlers. It was the one place where I could become one with nature and no other soul in the entire universe could find me.

I climbed to the top of the rock. With the sun filtering through the trees as it did the stained-glass windows of a church, I raised my arms up to the sky like an Indian and chanted a self-styled prayer thanking God for all of life. I felt closer to the Almighty than Pastor R. could ever lead me.

Back in the real world, my relationship with the spirit was a matter of debate. At home, my parents never asked a single question about the incident with Pastor R. I interpreted their silence as support. But three days later the school board met in an emergency session to debate the matter. Actually, their discussion concerned only the best form of punishment. They had no doubt I was wrong.

Fortunately, my favorite teacher, Mr. Wegmann, convinced the board to let me give my own version of the incident. I entered nervously. Once I began to speak, I stared directly at Pastor R. He sat with his head bowed and hands folded, the picture of piety. Afterward, I was told to go home and wait.

The next several days passed very slowly, and then one evening Mr. Wegmann came to our house after dinner. He informed my parents that I was officially excused from Pastor R.'s classes. No one was displeased. The light punishment implied that I had not acted improperly. Mr. Wegmann asked me what I thought. I replied that it struck me as fair, but before saying so officially I wanted one more condition met. I wanted Eva excused from Pastor R.'s class too. "Granted," said Mr. Wegmann.

45

For me, there was nothing more Godlike or inspiring of belief in some greater power than the outdoors. The highlight of my youth was unquestionably the time we spent in a little alpine cabin in Amden. The best guide, my father pointed out something about every flower and tree. We skied in the winter. Each summer, he led strenuous two-week hikes that taught us spartan living and strict discipline. He also let us explore the moors, meadows and brooks that ran through the forest.

But when my sister Erika lost her enthusiasm for these outings, we were concerned. By twelve years old, she had become increasingly uncomfortable going for hikes. On our annual school three-day hike, which was attended by several grown-ups and a teacher, she absolutely refused to participate. This should have been a red flag of something more serious. Having hiked long distances with my father with very little food or luxury, we were well trained for such trips. Even Eva and I could not understand what our sister's problem was. My father, who could not tolerate any "sissies," simply laid down the law and forced her to go anyway.

It was a mistake. Before leaving, she complained that her leg and hip hurt fiercely. On the first day out, she got very sick. One of the teachers and a parent brought her back home to Meilen where she was hospitalized, the start of years of abuse by doctors and hospitals. Although she was paralyzed on one side and limped on the other, nobody could make a diagnosis. She was in agony and pain to such an extent that very often when Eva and I came home from school, we could hear Erika screaming in the bedroom. Naturally this led to a lot of tiptoeing around the house and head-shaking over poor Erika.

Since no diagnosis could be verified, many people felt that this was hysteria or simply a way to get away from sports and physical activities. Years later, the obstetrician who delivered us made great efforts to find a diagnosis, which eventually turned out to be a cavity in the hipbone. In retrospect, she had poliomyelitis combined with osteomyelitis. In those days, that was difficult to diagnose. One of the orthopedic hospitals tortured her by forcing her on an escalator where she had to take long, painful steps. They thought if she exercised long enough, she would stop this "malingering."

I was frustrated at how my sister had to suffer. Thankfully, once a diagnosis was made and the proper treatment administered, Erika was able to go off to school in Zurich and live a good, productive and pain-free life. But I always felt a competent, caring physician could have done a lot more to help. Once, during Erika's hospitalizations, I wrote her a letter pledging my intention to become exactly that kind of doctor.

Of course, the world needed healing, and soon would need it even more. In 1939 the Nazi war machine was beginning to unleash its destructive force. Our teacher Mr. Wegmann, an officer in the Swiss Army, prepared us for the eventual outbreak of war. At home, my father entertained many German businessmen who reported on Hitler and said Jews were being rounded up in Poland and allegedly murdered in concentration camps, although no one knew for sure what was happening to them. But all the talk about war made us scared and uneasy.

One September morning my thrifty father came home with a radio, a luxury in our village. Suddenly, though, it was a necessity. Every night at seven-thirty, after dinner, we gathered around the large wooden box and listened to the reports of Nazi Germany's march through Poland. I sided with the brave Poles who were risking their lives to defend their homeland, and I cried when I heard descriptions of how the women and children of Warsaw were dying on the front lines. I bristled with anger when I heard reports that the Nazis were killing Jews. If I were a man I would have gone to fight.

But I was a young girl, not a man. So instead I promised God that when I became old enough I would travel to Poland and help those courageous souls defeat their oppressors. "As soon as I can," I whispered. "As soon as I can, I will go to Poland and help."

In the meantime, I hated the Nazis. I hated them even more when Swiss troopers confirmed the rumors about concentration camps for Jews. My own father and brother witnessed Nazi soldiers stationed along the Rhine machine-gun a human river of Jewish refugees as they attempted to cross into safety. Few made it to the Swiss side alive. Some were caught and sent to concentration camps. Many floated down the river dead. The atrocities were too great and too numerous to be hidden. Everyone I knew was outraged.

Each broadcast of news from the war sounded to me like a moral challenge. "No, we will never surrender," I shouted while listening to Winston Churchill. "Never!"

As the war raged, we learned the meaning of sacrifice. Refugees streamed across the Swiss borders. Food had to be rationed. My mother taught us how to put eggs away so they would keep for a year or two. Our lawns were turned into potato patches and vegetable gardens. Our basement contained so many canned goods it resembled a modern supermarket.

I took pride knowing I could survive on homegrown food, make my own bread, preserve fruits and vegetables and do without former luxuries. It was just a small contribution to the war effort, but it gave me a new confidence in being self-sufficient, and later on that would come in handy.

Given the conditions in neighboring countries, we had much to be grateful for. On a personal level, our lives were relatively undisturbed. At sixteen years of age, my sisters were preparing to be confirmed, a major event for a Swiss child. They studied with Pastor Zimmermann, a renowned Protestant minister, in Zurich. My family had a long association with him, and there was mutual love and respect. As the confirmation date neared, he confessed to my parents that he had dreamed about presiding over the confirmation of the Kübler triplets, which was a subtle way of asking, "What about Elisabeth?"

I had no intention of joining the church, but the pastor asked me to tell him all my criticisms of the church. I went through them one by one, from Pastor R. to my belief that no God, especially my notion of God, could be contained under any one roof or defined by man-made laws or conventions. "So why," I asked in an interested tone, "should I be part of such a church?"

Rather than try to change my mind, Pastor Zimmermann defended God and faith by arguing it was how people lived, not worshipped, that mattered. "Each day you must attempt to make the highest choices God offers," he said. "That is what truly determines if a person lives close to God."

I agreed, and so a few weeks after our talk, Pastor Zimmermann's dream came true. The Kübler triplets stood on a beautifully decorated stage inside his simple church as he towered over us and recited a verse from St. Paul's Epistle to the Corinthians: "And now abideth faith, hope, love, these three; but the greatest of these is love." Then Pastor Zimmermann faced us, raised a hand over our heads and upon each of us bestowed a single word as if it embodied us.

Eva was faith. Erika was hope. And I was love.

At a time when love seemed in short supply throughout the world, I accepted that as a gift, an honor and, above all else, a responsibility.

CHAPTER SIX

My Own Lab Coat

❧

By the time my public schooling ended in spring 1942, I had become a mature and thoughtful young adult. Deep thoughts resided in my head. My future, as far as I was concerned, was medical school. My desire to become a doctor was as strong as ever. I literally felt called to the profession. What was better than healing the sick, giving hope to the hopeless and comforting those in pain?

But my father was still in charge, and the night when he turned his thoughts to the future of his three daughters was no different than it had been that tumultuous night in the family kitchen. He sent Eva to finishing school and Erika on to gymnasium in Zurich. As for me, my father again assigned me to become the secretary/bookkeeper for his business. He showed little insight into me by explaining what a wonderful opportunity he was providing for me. "The door is wide open," he said.

I did not attempt to hide my disappointment and made it clear that I would never ever accept a prison sentence like that. I had a creative, thoughtful intellect and a restless nature. I would die sitting at a desk every day.

My father angered quickly. He was not interested in debate, especially with a child. What did a child know?

"If my offer is not suitable, then you can go away and work as a maid," he huffed.

A tense silence took over the dining room. I did not want to fight with my father, but every fiber in my body refused to accept the future that he had chosen for me. I considered the option he gave me. I certainly did not want to work as a maid, but I wanted to be the one who made the decisions regarding my future.

"I will work as a maid," I said, and as soon as I did my father walked into his study and slammed the door.

The next day my mother saw an ad in the newspaper. The French-speaking widow of a wealthy professor in Romilly, a village on Lake Geneva, sought help caring for her home, three children, pets and garden. I got the job and left a week later. My sisters were so upset they did not see me off. At the train station, I struggled with an old leather suitcase almost as large as I was. Before departing, my mother gave me a wide-brimmed hat to go along with my wool suit and then asked me to reconsider. Even though I was already homesick, I was too stubborn to change my mind. I had made *my* decision.

I regretted it as soon as I got off the train and said hello to my new boss, Madame Perret, and her three children. I had spoken in Schweizer-deutsch (Swiss German). She took immediate offense. "We speak only in French," she said. "Starting right now." Madame was a large, heavy woman with a nasty temper. She had once served as the professor's housekeeper, but after his wife died she married him. Then he died. She inherited everything except his pleasant disposition.

That was my bad luck. I worked from 6 A.M. to midnight every day, with a half day off two weekends per month. I began by waxing the floors in the morning and polishing the silver and then I shopped, cooked, served meals and straightened up into the evening. At midnight, Madame usually wanted a cup of tea. Finally I was permitted to go to my little room. Usually I fell asleep before my head hit the pillow.

But if Madame did not hear the floor-waxing machine going in the living room by six-thirty she pounded on my door. "Time to start!"

In my letters home, I never admitted that I was hungry and miserable, especially as the weather turned cold and the holidays approached. As Christmas neared, I was desperately homesick. I grew sad remembering the sounds of my entire family singing joyous holiday songs at the piano. I pictured the arts and crafts my sisters and I made for each other. Madame just made me work harder, though. She entertained constantly and then prohibited me from looking at their Christmas tree. "Only family," she said scornfully, a tone that was echoed by her children, who were not much younger than I.

I hit a low point the night she had a holiday dinner party for her husband's former university colleagues. Per Madame's order, I served asparagus as an appetizer and hurried into the dining room to clear the plates as soon as she rang the bell alerting me that her guests were finished. But when I entered, I saw the asparagus was still on everyone's plate. So I turned around and left. Madame rang the bell again. The same scene was repeated. And then it happened a third time. It would have been comical if I did not think I was losing my mind.

Finally Madame stormed into the kitchen. How could I be so stupid? "Get in there and take those plates out," she said, fuming. "Educated people only eat the tips of the asparagus. The rest is left on the plate!" Maybe so, but after I cleared the plates I devoured what was left of the uneaten asparagus. It tasted as delicious as it looked. As I swallowed the final spear, one of Madame's guests came in, a professor, who asked what in the world I was doing there.

I told him I was starving and had practically no money. "The reason I'm sticking it out a whole year is that I need to be old enough to enter a laboratory," I said with tears welling in my tired eyes. "I want to train as a lab technician so that I can go on to medical school."

The professor listened sympathetically. Then he handed me his card and promised to help me find a job in a suitable lab. He also offered temporary lodging at his home in Lausanne and said he would tell his wife as soon as he got back home. In exchange, I had to promise to leave this dreadful place.

Before Christmas, I had a half day off. I went to Lausanne and knocked on the professor's door. The professor's wife answered and sadly informed me that her husband had died a few days earlier. We talked for a long time. She said that he had even looked for a lab job for me, but she did not know where. I left even more depressed.

Back at Madame's, I worked harder than ever. By Christmas Eve, she had filled the house with guests. I was constantly busy cooking, planning, cleaning and doing laundry. One evening I begged Madame for a look at the Christmas tree. Just five minutes. I needed to recharge spiritually. "No, it's not Christmas yet," she said, aghast, and then she reiterated her previous admonition: "Besides, this is for family. Not employees." Right then, I decided to leave. Anyone who would not share their Christmas tree was not worthy of my work and care.

After borrowing a straw suitcase from a girl I knew in Vevey, I plotted my escape. When the floor-waxing machine failed to whir as usual on Christmas morning, Madame came into my room and ordered me to start work. But rather than comply, I boldly informed her that I had stopped waxing the floors permanently. Then I grabbed my stuff, threw it on a sled and raced to catch the first train out of town. I stayed overnight in Geneva with a friend, who pampered me with a bubble bath, tea, sandwiches and pastries, and then loaned me money to get the rest of the way home to Meilen.

I arrived home the day after Christmas. I slipped my skinny body through the milk box and headed straight for the kitchen. I knew my family would be away in the mountains for their traditional holiday getaway, so I was pleasantly surprised when I heard a noise upstairs and it turned out to be my sister Erika, whose impaired leg had caused her to stay behind. She was just as startled and happy to discover the sounds she heard downstairs came from me. We spent the entire night sitting on her bed, catching up on our lives.

I told the same stories the next day to my parents, who were angry that I had been hungry and exploited. They wondered why I had not come home sooner. My explanation did not please my father, but given what I had been through, he tempered his anger and let me enjoy a comfortable bed and nourishing meals.

When my sisters went back to school, I faced the same old problem of my future. Once again my father offered me a job at his business. But this time he added another option, one that showed a lot of personal growth on his part. He said that if I did not want to work there, I could find a job that I wanted, a job that would make me happy. That was the best news of my young life, and I prayed I would find something.

A few days later, my mother heard about an opening in a new

biochemical research institute. The lab was located in Feldmeiler, a few miles from Meilen, and it sounded perfect. I made an appointment to meet the lab's owner and dressed up for the interview, trying hard to look older and professional. But Dr. Hans Braun, an ambitious young scientist, could not have cared less. He appeared frantically busy and said he needed smart people to work right away. "Can you start now?" he asked.

"Yes," I said.

I was hired as an apprentice.

"There's just one requirement," he said. "Bring your own white lab coat."

It was the one thing I did not have. My heart sank. I feared opportunity slipping, and I guess it showed.

"If you don't have one, I'll be glad to supply one," said Dr. Braun.

I was ecstatic then, and even happier when I arrived for work Monday morning at eight and saw three wonderful white lab coats, with my name embroidered on them, hanging on the door of my laboratory. There could not have been a happier human on the planet.

Half of Dr. Braun's laboratory was devoted to manufacturing creams and cosmetics and lotions, while the side where I worked was a large greenhouse designed for researching the effect of cancerous materials on plants. Dr. Braun theorized that cancer-causing agents could be accurately and inexpensively tested on plants rather than on animals. His enthusiasm made his notions seem more than plausible. After a while I noticed he sometimes came to the lab depressed and skeptical of everything and everyone and spent the day hiding behind locked doors. Later I realized he was a manic-depressive. But his arching mood swings never interfered with my duties, which included injecting certain plants with nutritious substances, others with carcinogens, and then keeping strict observations in ledger books about which ones grew normally, excessively, abnormally or just plain poorly.

Not only was I swept up in the importance of the work, which had the possibility of saving lives, but I received lessons in chemistry and science from a friendly lab technician who indulged my limitless appetite to learn. After a few months, I began traveling to Zurich two days a week for classes in chemistry, physics and math, and topping thirty male classmates with straight A's. The number two grade point average belonged to another girl. But after nine months of bliss my dream turned into a nightmare when Dr. Braun, who had spent millions opening the lab, went bankrupt.

None of us knew until we showed up for work one August morning and found the office closed. Dr. Braun's fate was as unclear as his whereabouts. Either he was hospitalized for one of his manic episodes or he was in jail. Who knew when we would see him again, and it turned out the answer was never. Meanwhile, police officers outside informed us that we were dismissed, but generously gave us time to clean up the lab and save pertinent data. After a bunch of us shared a sad goodbye tea, I walked through the door at home freshly unemployed and profoundly crushed that yet another dream had been shattered.

As a result of my bad luck, I found the key to my future career. When I woke in the morning, I had only to imagine working at my father's office in order to stop pitying myself and begin looking for a job. My father gave me three whole weeks to look for new employment. If I did not find anything by then, I had to start as his bookkeeper, a fate I could not conceive of after the happiness of working in a research lab. Wasting no time, I got the Zurich telephone book and wrote with a feverish intensity to every research institute, hospital and clinic. In addition to including my grades, letters of recommendation and a photo, I pleaded for a quick response.

It was the end of summer, not a particularly good time to be looking for a job. I ran to the mailbox every day. Each day felt like a year. The earliest responses were not favorable. Nor were those that came during the second week. All of them admired my enthusiasm, my love of their work and my grades, but their quotas for apprenticeships were already filled. They encouraged me to reapply the next year. Then they would be happy to consider me. But that was too late.

For nearly a week I waited by the mailbox each day without luck. Then toward the end of the week, the mailman delivered the letter I had prayed for. The dermatology department at Canton Hospital in Zurich had just lost one of its lab apprentices and needed to fill the vacancy quickly. I wasted no time getting there. Doctors and nurses hustled down the corridors. I breathed the distinct scent of medicine common to all hospitals as if it was my first breath, and I felt right at home.

The dermatology department's lab was in the hospital's basement. It was run by Dr. Karl Zehnder, whose windowless office was stuck in a corner. I could tell Dr. Zehnder worked very hard. There were papers all over his desk and the lab itself buzzed with work. After a good interview, Dr. Zehnder hired me. I could not wait to tell my father. I also got a great measure of satisfaction telling Dr. Zehnder that when I started on Monday morning I would bring my own lab coat.

My Promise

Every day I walked into the hospital I breathed what to me was the most sacred, holy, most wonderful smell in the whole wide world, and then hurried down to my windowless laboratory. In this strange, chaotic time of war, when basics like food and doctors were in short supply, I knew that I would not be stuck in the basement forever, and I was right.

After several weeks on the job, Dr. Zehnder asked if I was interested in taking blood samples from real live patients. The patients from whom I would be taking the samples were prostitutes in the later-stage symptoms of venereal disease. In those days, before penicillin, VD sufferers were treated like AIDS patients would be in the 1980s—they were feared, abandoned, shunned, locked away. Later Dr. Zehnder admitted that he expected me to say no. Instead I marched right into the dismal ward.

I think that is what separates those who are called into the healing profession and those who do it for the money.

The patients were all in super-bad shape. Their bodies were so grossly infected with disease that most could not even sit in a chair or lie in their beds. Instead they were suspended from hammocks. On first sight, they were pathetic, suffering creatures. But they were human beings, and once I spoke to them I found the majority to be terribly warm, nice, caring people who had been discarded by their families and by society. They had nothing, which made me want to help even more.

After taking their blood, I sat on their beds and talked for hours about their lives, the things they had seen and experienced and existence in general. I realized they had emotional needs that were every bit as dire as their physical requirements. They craved friendship and compassion, which I could provide, and in return they opened my heart as wide as my eyes. It was a fair exchange that prepared me for worse.

On June 6, 1944, Allied troops landed in Normandy. D-Day. It changed the war, and pretty soon we felt the effects of the massive invasion. Refugees streamed into Switzerland. They came in waves. For days. Hundreds at a time. They marched, limped, crawled and were carried. Some came from as far away as France. Some were injured old men. Most were women and children. Virtually overnight our hospital overflowed with these traumatized victims.

They were led directly into the dermatology ward, where we put them in our large bathhouse and deloused and disinfected them. Without even asking my boss for permission, I worked directly on the children. I smeared them with liquid soap to take care of their scabies and rubbed them with a soft brush. After they dressed in freshly washed clothing, I dispensed what I felt they needed most, hugs and soothing words. "Everything will be all right," I said.

This went on nonstop for three weeks. I completely lost myself in the necessary work and gave little thought to my own well-being when others were so much worse. Meals became afterthoughts. Sleep? Who had time? I crawled home after midnight and started again the next day at dawn. I was so focused on the suffering, frightened children, so out of the normal daily loop, so involved with responsibilities other than those I had originally been hired to do at the lab, that I was several days behind what should have been big news: my boss, Dr. Zehnder, left and was replaced by Dr. Abraham Weitz.

I was too busy trying to find enough food for the famished refugees. With help from another lab apprentice, a rascal named Baldwin, who had a taste for stirring up mischief, we came up with a plan to fill those growling stomachs. For several nights in a row, we ordered hundreds of complete meals from the hospital kitchen, picked them up with large carts and distributed them to the children. If any was left over, we fed the adults. Eventually, after children and adults alike were cleaned, clothed and fed, they were taken to various schoolhouses in the city and handed over to the Red Cross.

Inevitably, I knew our diversion of precious food supplies would be detected and result in disciplinary action. I just hoped it would not be too severe when Dr. Weitz summoned me into his office, but I expected to be fired. In addition to the food, I had completely forgotten to excuse myself from my lab work, not to mention greeting my new boss. But instead of chewing me out, Dr. Weitz complimented me. He had, he admitted, watched me from afar as I worked with the children and had never seen anyone as consumed by or as happy with their work. "You must take care of refugee children," he said. "That is your destiny."

I could not have felt more relieved or inspired. Then Dr. Weitz continued to tell me about the urgent need for medical care in his native country, war-torn Poland. His horrifying stories, especially those of Jewish children in concentration camps, moved me to tears. His own family had suffered greatly. "They need people like you there," he said. "If you can, if you finish your apprenticeship, you must promise me that you will go to Poland and help me with this work there." Grateful at not being fired, and also inspired, I promised.

But then the other shoe dropped. That night the hospital's chief administrator called me and Baldwin to his office. Droopy with fatigue, I had nothing but disdain for this spoiled, fat, self-contented bureaucrat who sat behind a large mahogany desk, puffing a cigar and looking at the two of us lowly lab technicians as if we were thieves. He demanded that we repay the cost of the hundreds of meals we served the refugee children or come up with an equivalent amount in rationing coupons. "If not," he said, "you will be subject to immediate termination."

I was devastated, since I did not want to lose my job and apprenticeship, but I had no access to that kind of money. Down in the basement, Dr. Weitz sensed something was drastically wrong and got me to confess. He shook his head in disgust and told me not to worry about the bureaucracy. The next day he went to the leaders of Zurich's Jewish community and with their help the hospital was quickly repaid for the unauthorized meals with a large number of ration cards. Not only did I get to keep my job; I reaffirmed the promise I had made to my benefactor, Dr. Weitz, to help rebuild Poland once the war ended. I just had no idea how soon that would be.

*   *   *

Countless times in years past I had helped my father prepare our mountain cabin in Amden for visitors, but it was different when he asked me to go there with him in early January 1945. For one thing, I needed the weekend rest. But he also promised the visitors were going to be people I would really enjoy, and he was right. Our guests were from the International Voluntary Service for Peace. They numbered twenty in all, and were, to me, a group of mostly young, smart idealists from all parts of Europe. After lots of joyous singing, laughter and ravenous eating, I listened raptly as various members explained how the IVSP—founded after World War I and later a model for the American Peace Corps—was dedicated to creating world peace and cooperation.

World peace? Cooperation among nations and people? Assisting the ravaged and devastated people of Europe once the war ended? These people were describing my greatest dreams. Their stories of humanitarian work were music to my soul. Once I discovered there was a branch office in Zurich, I thought of little else other than signing up. And as soon as it appeared the war might end soon, I filled out an application and imagined myself leaving the peaceful island of Switzerland to help the survivors of the war-devastated countries in Europe.

Talk about music for the soul. There was no greater symphony than the sound that filled the outdoors on May 7, 1945—the day the war in Europe ended. I was at the hospital. As if on cue but quite spontaneously, the bells in the churches throughout Switzerland began to ring. All at the same time, making the air resonate with the jubilant chimes of victory and, most of all, peace. Helped by several hospital workers, I took patient after patient, including those too weak to get out of bed, up to the roof, where they could join in the celebration.

It was a moment everyone from the old and weak to the new-born shared in equally. Some stood, others sat. Still others were in wheelchairs or lying on stretchers, some suffering intense pain. But right then it did not matter. We were stitched together by

62

love and hope, the essence of human existence, and it was, to my mind, quite beautiful and unforgettable. Unfortunately, it was just an illusion.

Anyone who thought life was back to normal had only to join the IVSP. A few days after the celebrating ended, I heard from the leader of a contingent of fifty or so volunteers who planned to enter the newly opened borders of France and rebuild Ecurcey, a small, once-picturesque country village that had been almost totally destroyed by the Nazis. They wanted me to join them. I could hardly imagine a better fortune than to drop everything and go, though so much had to be done before I could.

There was my job, of course. But Dr. Weitz, my biggest supporter, instantly gave me a leave from the hospital. Home was a different story. When I raised the issue at the dinner table, more as a fait accompli than a request for permission, my father burst out that I was nuts. Also naive about all the hazards I faced there. My mother, pondering my sisters' more predictable futures, no doubt wished I could be more like them rather than face dangers such as land mines, food shortages and diseases. But none of them understood my obsession. My destiny, whatever it turned out to be, was still many miles ahead, somewhere in the desert of human suffering.

If I was ever to get there, if I was ever to help, I had to get on the path.

CHAPTER EIGHT

A Sense of Purpose

❧

I looked like a teenager going to camp as I rode an old bicycle someone had found across the border into Ecurcey. It was my first time outside the safety of the Swiss borders, and I got a fast education in the tragedy the war left behind. Ecurcey, a quaint hamlet before the war, was completely destroyed. Homes were razed. A few young men, all with injuries, wandered around aimlessly. The remaining population was mostly old people, women, a handful of children and a group of Nazi prisoners being held in the schoolhouse basement.

Our arrival was a big event. The whole town turned out, including the mayor. "I have never been more grateful," he said.

I felt the same way—grateful for the chance to serve people who needed assistance. The whole group of IVSP workers clicked with vitality. Everything I had learned up to then, from basic survival skills my father had taught me on our mountain hikes to the rudiments of medicine I had picked up in the hospital, was quickly put to use. The work was tremendously rewarding. Each day had a sense of purpose.

Our living conditions were abysmal, yet I had never been happier. We slept on broken bunks or on the ground under the stars. If it rained, we got wet. Our tools consisted of picks, axes and shovels. An older woman among us—she was in her sixties— recalled tales of having done similar work after World War I in 1918. She made us feel blessed for the little we did have.

As the younger of two female volunteers, I was appointed

cook. Since none of the buildings that stood had viable kitchens, several of us created one outdoors using a huge wood-burning stove. Food was a big problem. Our own rations disappeared almost immediately from portioning them out to the whole village, and there was nothing in the local grocery store, which was miraculously intact, except for dust on the shelves. Often it took several volunteers the whole day just to scour the nearby woods and farms for enough food for a single meal. Once a single dried fish was supposed to feed fifty.

But we made up for our lack of meat, potatoes and butter with spirited camaraderie. At night we shared stories and sang songs, which, I discovered, were enjoyed by the German prisoners in the school basement. When we first got to Ecurcey, we noticed the prisoners were taken to the outlying fields every morning and forced to walk over the entire area. At sundown, one or two fewer prisoners returned. Upon inquiring, we learned they were being used as human minesweepers. The ones who did not come back had been blown up by mines they had planted. Outraged, we stopped the practice by threatening to walk in front of them and instead had them do construction work.

With the exception of the local villagers, no one there hated the Nazis more than I did. If the crimes they had committed in this very village were not enough to stir my enmity, I had only to think about Dr. Weitz at the lab wondering if any of his family back in Poland were still alive. But over my first weeks there I saw these soldiers as human beings, defeated, demoralized, hungry, frightened of being blown to bits in their own minefields, and my heart opened up.

Instead of Nazis, I saw them simply as needy men. At night, I slipped them little bars of soap or pencils and paper through the iron shutters on the basement windows. They in turn poured their hearts out in very moving letters that I stuffed in my clothes and forwarded to their families once I got back home. Years later, the families of those soldiers, most of whom made it back alive, sent me the most appreciative thank-yous. In fact, the month I spent in Ecurcey, despite the trials, despite being heartbroken when I had to go back home, could not have been more positive. We rebuilt many homes, yes. But the best thing we gave those people was love and hope.

In return, they confirmed our belief that this was important work. On my way out, the mayor bid me farewell and an ailing old man who had made friends with all the volunteers but knew me best as "the little cook" handed me a note that said, "You have rendered the greatest humanitarian service. I write to you because I have no family of my own. I want to tell you that no matter whether we live or whether we die here, we shall never forget you. Please accept a deep, heartfelt thank-you and love from one human being to another."

In my quest to figure out who I was and what I wanted to do in life, this message was the sort that helped. The evil of Nazi Germany was punished during the war and continued to be brought to trial afterward. But I realized the wounds inflicted by the war, the residual suffering and pain that were experienced in virtually every home, just as with today's problems of violence, homelessness and AIDS, could not be healed unless people like me, like the IVSP, recognized the moral imperative to pitch in and help.

Changed by that experience, I found the prosperity of my Swiss home hard to take. There was such abundance. I had trouble reconciling shops full of food and successful businesses with the hurt and ruin in the rest of Europe. But I was needed at home too. Having injured his hip, my father was in the process of selling our home and moving to an apartment closer to his office in Zurich. With my sisters studying in Europe and my brother in India, I packed our belongings and took care of other details.

Emotionally, I was very mixed. Sadly, I realized this was good-bye to my youth, to those glorious walks through the vineyards and dances on my private sun rock in the meadow. At the same time, I had grown up quite a bit and was ready to move into the next stage. Briefly, I went back to work in the hospital's lab. In June, I passed my apprenticeship exam, and the following month I landed a spectacular research job in the ophthalmology department at the University of Zurich. But my boss, Professor Marc Amsler, a famous physician, who gave me extraordinary responsibilities that included assisting him in surgery, knew I did not plan on staying more than a year. Not only was I studying for medical school; I still had the IVSP on my mind.

And the promise I made to Dr. Weitz. Yes, Poland was still in my plan.

"Ah, the swallow must fly again," said Dr. Amsler when I gave notice at the hospital after the IVSP called with a new assignment. He was not angry or disappointed. For the past year, he had anticipated my departure, since we had often spoken of my commitment to the IVSP. There was, I noted, a twinkle of envy in his eyes. Mine held the promise of new adventure.

It was spring. The IVSP had promised to help the people in a polluted coal-mining town outside Mons in Belgium construct a playground on a mountain above the dirty, dusty air. It was, I learned, a commitment made before the war. The chief of the Zurich office explained I could have train passage as far as the tracks went, which was only partway, but I assured them that I could hitchhike the whole way by myself. Traveling through Paris, which I had never seen before, I lugged my stuffed rucksack in and out of various youth hostels till I arrived in the grimy coal-mining town.

It was a depressing place where the dirt filled the air and coated everything a dull and dusty grayish yuck. Thanks to horrible side effects like black-lung disease, the life expectancy there averaged barely more than forty years, which was not much of a future for the village's lovely children. Our task, and the town's dream, was to clear one of the mountains of coal-mining debris and build a playground in the clean air above the polluted muck. Using shovels and picks, we worked till our muscles ached with exhaustion, but the villagers offered us so much pie and pastry that I gained eight pounds in the few weeks I was there.

I also gained important contacts. One night as a bunch of us sang folk songs after a hearty dinner, I met the one American in our group. He was a youngish man, one of several Quakers. He understood my broken English and said his name was David Richie. "From New Jersey." But I already knew of his reputation. Richie was among the most famous volunteers, a truly dedicated peacenik. His work had taken him from the Philadelphia ghettos to the worst postwar sites in Europe and, most recently, he explained, in Poland. He was, he added, about to go back there.

Oh my God! Here was proof that nothing happened by accident.

Poland.

Seizing the opportunity, I told Richie about the promise I had made to my previous boss and begged him to take me along. He agreed that help was drastically needed, but suggested getting me there would be quite difficult. Safe, reliable transportation was virtualy nonexistent. Money for good tickets was not available. Though I was small compared with most, and looked much younger than twenty and had about fifteen dollars in my pocket, I paid no attention to such obstacles. "I will hitchhike!" I exclaimed. Impressed, amused and aware of the value of passion, Richie said he would try to get me there.

No promises. But he would try.

It almost did not matter. The night before I left for a new assignment in Sweden, I incurred a severe burn while cooking dinner. An old cast-iron pan snapped in two, splattering hot oil on my leg. It caused third-degree burns and blisters. Heavily bandaged, I set off anyway with some clean underwear and a wool blanket in case I needed to sleep outdoors. By Hamburg, though, my leg was throbbing with pain. When I removed the bandages, I saw that it was severely infected. Fearing I would get stuck in Germany, which was the last place I wanted to be, I found a doctor who treated my wound with some ointment that enabled me to keep going.

It was still a struggle. But thanks to a Red Cross volunteer who saw me in anguish on the train, I hobbled into a fully equipped hospital in Denmark. Several days of treatment and delicious food gave me the capacity to be my old self at the IVSP camp in Stockholm. But being thickheaded also has its downside. Now healthy and replenished, I was frustrated by my assignment— training a group of young German men to run their own IVSP camps. The work lacked challenge. Plus I was turned off by most of these guys, who admitted they had supported Hitler's Nazis rather than take a moral stand against them, as I argued they should have. I suspected they were opportunists grabbing three good meals a day in Sweden.

But there were some fantastic people. One ninety-three-year-old Russian émigré fell in love with me. He nurtured me through weeks of homesickness and provided interesting conversation about Russia and Poland. As my twenty-first birthday came and went, he brightened my days by taking the journal I carried with me and writing, "Your shining eyes reminded me of sunshine. My hope is that we'll meet again and that we'll have the opportunity to greet the sun together. Au revoir." If I ever needed a boost, I just turned to that page.

Having made an impression, that kind-spirited man vanished. Life was dominated by such randomness. I realized that you just had to be open to its significance. Did something happen to him? Or did he know that our time was up? As soon as he left, a telegram arrived from my IVSP friend David Richie. I opened it anxiously and felt the electricity of anticipation that comes when all your hopes and dreams are suddenly confirmed. "Peterli, come to Poland as soon as possible," Richie wrote. "Greatly needed." Finally, I thought. No birthday present could have been any better.

CHAPTER NINE

Blessed Soil

❧

Getting to Warsaw was difficult. I cut hay and milked cows for a farmer to earn enough money for the journey. Before leaving Stockholm, I got a visa and spent nearly all my hard-earned cash on a boat ticket. Some boat, though. The ship's hull was rusted and its nonstop creaking did not inspire confidence that we would make it to Gdansk. My passage was no-frills. At night, I curled up on a rough wooden bench and dreamed of luxuries like a warm blanket and comfy pillow, and I ignored the four guys who roamed the deck near me in the darkness. I was too tired to worry.

As it turned out, there was no need. In the morning the four men, all of whom were from different Eastern European countries, introduced themselves as doctors. They were returning from a medical conference. Fortunately for me, they suggested I join them on the rest of the journey to Warsaw. The train station was jammed, and the platform outside, where the train actually stopped, was worse. Not only was it crowded with people with enormous amounts of luggage but there were people carrying chickens and geese, others leading goats and sheep, like a chaotic Noah's ark.

If I had been by myself, I never would have gotten on the train. When it arrived, something close to pandemonium broke out as people clamored to board. One of the doctors, a tall, lanky Hungarian, jumped up on the roof with the agility of a monkey and then pulled the rest of us up there with him. I grabbed on to the chimney just as the whistle blew and the train began rolling down the tracks. It was not the most secure seating, especially going through tunnels, when we had to lie down flat on our stomachs, or when the smoke billowed out of the chimney in chunky black clouds that made each breath a struggle. But after the train emptied out a bit, we got our own compartment. As we shared food and exchanged life stories, the trip suddenly seemed downright luxurious.

Getting to Warsaw was an adventure, but actually arriving there was beyond belief. For my traveling companions, it was where they changed trains. I, on the other hand, knew I was at a crossroads, the place where something was destined to happen. With our faces blackened by soot like a bunch of chimney sweeps, we said goodbye. Then I scanned the crowd for signs of my American Quaker friend. I had not been able to tell anyone when I was arriving. How would they know when to pick me up? Where was I supposed to go?

But fate is a lot like faith; both require fervent belief in God's will. I looked one way, then another. No sign of anyone. Then from out of the crowd I saw a large Swiss flag rise above the sea of people. Then I saw Richie, who had come there on a hunch, and several others. It was a miracle they were there. Boy, did I give him a hug. His friends offered hot tea and soup. Food had never tasted as good as it did then. A long sleep in a nice bed would have been welcome too. But we climbed into the back of a flatbed truck and spent the remainder of the day driving over bumpy, unpaved, bombed-out roads to the IVSP camp in Lucima, a fertile farming area.

That road trip offered evidence of how desperately we were needed. Almost two years after the war ended, Warsaw was still in ruins. Whole blocks of buildings were transformed into mountains of rubble. The city's population, which numbered some 300,000, hid in underground homes, the only sign of human life coming at night when wisps of smoke rose from open fires used for cooking and warmth. The outlying villages, destroyed by the Germans and Russians, were in similarly horrendous shape. Entire families just dug in, like burrowing animals. In the countryside, trees were mowed down and the ground cratered from bombings.

Rolling into Lucima, I felt blessed to be among those strong

72

enough to help the many villagers in dire need of medical care. Was it possible to feel any other way? No, not when there was no local hospital or medical facility and you were among people struggling amid various stages of typhoid and tuberculosis. The lucky ones merely endured old, infected shrapnel wounds. Children were dying from common diseases like measles. But despite their problems, they were wonderful, generous people.

You did not have to be an expert in disaster relief to see the only way to deal with a situation like this was to simply roll up your sleeves and start to work. The IVSP camp consisted of three huge tents. I slept most nights outside, under the wool military blanket that kept me warm throughout my travels in Europe. Once again, I was appointed cook. Nothing made me happier than to turn canisters of dried bananas, some donated geese, flour and eggs and whatever other ingredients happened to be available into tasty meals that would please these volunteers who came from all over the globe united by a single purpose.

By the time of my arrival, a number of homes had been rebuilt and a brand-new schoolhouse was under construction. I worked as a mason, bricklayer and roofer. My Polish was spotty, but each morning I was tutored, while washing my clothes in the river, by a painfully thin young woman who was dying of leukemia. Having witnessed so much pain and misery in her brief lifetime, she did not consider her own situation the worst disaster in the world. Far from it. Somehow she accepted her fate without any bitterness or blame. To her, it was simply her life, at least a part of it. Needless to say, she taught me more than a new language.

Each day you had to be a jack-of-all-trades. Once I helped pacify the mayor and a group of local VIPs who were up in arms because we had built without official permits—meaning no pay-offs to them. Another time I helped a farmer's cow give birth. The tasks could be anything, and they usually were. One afternoon I was laying bricks at the schoolhouse when a man fell and ripped a huge gash in his leg. Under normal circumstances, the injury would have required stitches. But there was no one around other than me and a Polish woman, who quickly scooped up a handful of soil and plastered it over the wound. I leapt off the roof, screaming, "No, it will cause an infection!"

Despite my concern, the local healers were like shamans. They practiced an old, earthy folk medicine, like homeopathy, and knew exactly what they were doing.

Still, they were impressed when I tied up the leg to stop the bleeding. From then on, they referred to me as "Pani Doctor." I tried explaining otherwise, but no one could tell them any different, including me.

Up till then, all the medical needs were handled by two women, Hanka and Danka. They were forthright, fabulous women, or *Feldschers,* as they were called. Both of them had served with the Polish Resistance on the Russian front, where they had trained in basic field medicine and seen every possible kind of wound, injury, sickness and horror. Needless to say, they were not timid about anything.

Once they heard how I had stopped the man's leg from bleeding, they asked about my background. As soon as they heard the word "hospital," they embraced me as one of them. From then on, they brought the sick and injured to the construction site for me to examine. I mean patients with everything from simple infections to limbs that needed amputating. I did what I could to help, though often it was nothing more than a good hug.

Then one day they gave me an incredible gift. It was a two-room log cabin. They had cleaned it up, put in a wood-burning stove and shelves and decided it would be a medical clinic where the three of us could treat patients. My construction work ended right there.

I do not know if what I did next was practice medicine or pray for miracles. Every morning twenty-five to thirty people lined up outside the clinic. Some had walked for days. Often they waited for hours. If it was raining, they were allowed to wait in the room we normally reserved for the geese, chickens, goats and other contributions people made to our camp in lieu of money. The other room was used for surgery. We had few instruments, little medicine and no anesthesia. Remarkably, though, we performed many brave and intricate surgeries. We removed limbs. We took out shrapnel. We delivered babies. One day a pregnant woman showed up with a tumor the size of a grapefruit. We opened it up, drained the pus and tried our best to remove the lump. After we assured her that her baby would be okay, she got up and walked home.

There was no end to the resiliency of these people. Their

74

courage and will to live made a strong impression on me. At times, I suspected that determination alone was responsible for their high rate of recovery. The essence of their existence, I realized, and of every living creature, was simply to go on, to survive. For someone who had once written that her goal was to figure out the meaning of life, this was a most profound lesson in life and living.

My biggest test came one night when Hanka and Danka rushed to emergencies in neighboring villages and left me in charge of the clinic. It was my first time flying solo. And what a time. We were completely out of medical supplies. If something happened, I would have to improvise. Fortunately, the day was quiet and the night was seductively pleasant. I rolled out my blanket and said to myself, "Ah, nothing's going to wake me up tonight. For once, I will get a good night's sleep."

But that was like a jinx. About midnight I heard what sounded like the whimper of a small child. I refused to open my eyes. Maybe I was dreaming. And if not, then so what? Ordinarily patients arrived at all hours every night. If I answered all of them, I never would have slept a moment. So I pretended to sleep.

But then I heard it again. A small child's whimper. A helpless, pleading cry that didn't let up. Then a raspy breath, an agonizing gasp for air.

Hating myself for being such a softy, I opened my eyes. As I feared, I was not dreaming. Illuminated by the soft light of a full moon, a peasant woman sat beside me. She had wrapped herself in a blanket. Surely the cries were not coming from her. As I sat up, I heard the whimper-rasp again and saw she was cradling a little child in her arms. I studied the child as best I could while my eyes adjusted to being awake—it was a little boy, I noted—and then switched my gaze to his mother. She apologized for waking me up so late but said she had walked from her own village after hearing about the lady doctors who made sick people healthy again.

I put my hand to the boy's forehead. About three years old, he burned with a high fever. I also noted blisters around his lips and tongue and the look of dehydration. Signs of one thing—typhoid. Unfortunately, there was little I could do. There was no medication, I explained with a sorry shrug. Nothing. I said, "The only thing I can do is take you into the clinic and make a cup of hot tea." Appreciative, she followed me into the cabin. As her child labored to breathe, she stared at me as only a mother can. Quietly. Sadly. Pleading with dark black eyes that reflected unimaginable depths of sorrow. "You have to save him," she said matter-of-factly.

I shook my head in resignation.

"No, you have to save this last child," she continued. Then, without a tremor of emotion, she explained, "He is the last of my thirteen children. The others all perished in Maidanek, the concentration camp. But this one was born there. I don't want him to die now that we have made it out."

Even if this little clinic had been a fully equipped hospital, it was unlikely the child could be saved. But I hated to sound like a helpless fool. This woman had already suffered enough cruelty. If she had somehow clung to hope while her entire family had been murdered in the gas chambers, then I could also summon the strength within myself. So I thought my brains out for a moment and came up with a plan. There was a hospital in Lublin, the next city over. Though the camp could not provide trans-portation, we could walk. If the child survived the trip, perhaps we could persuade the hospital to admit him.

The plan was risky. But the woman, knowing it was the only option, scooped the boy in her arms and said, "Okay, let's go."

Through the night, we talked and alternated carrying the boy, who was not doing well. At sunup we reached the tall iron gates outside the massive stone hospital. They were locked, and a guard said no more patients were being admitted. Had we walked all these miles for nothing? I looked at the listless boy fading in and out of consciousness. No, this effort would not be in vain. The moment I spotted someone who looked like he might be a doctor, I grabbed his attention. Reluctantly, he felt the child, took his pulse and then concluded he was hopeless. "We already have people on beds in the bathrooms," the doctor said. "Since he doesn't have a chance, there's no point to taking him in."

Suddenly, I became an angry, aggressive woman. "I'm from Switzerland," I said, moving directly under his nose. "I walked and hitchhiked to Poland to help the Polish people. I'm taking care of fifty patients a day in a tiny clinic in Lucima by myself. Now I've just walked all this way to save this child. If you don't admit him, I will go back to Switzerland and tell everybody the Poles are the most hard-hearted people, that they have no love or compassion, and that a Polish doctor had no empathy for a woman whose child, the last of thirteen, survived a concentration camp."

That did it. Grudgingly, the doctor reached for the child and agreed to admit him, but under one condition: both the child's mother and I had to leave him there for three weeks. "In three weeks either the boy will be buried or he will be well enough to be taken back," the doctor said. Without pausing to think, the mother blessed her child and relinquished him to the doctor. She had done as much as was humanly possible and I sensed her relief as doctor and child disappeared into the hospital. After there was no more for us to see, I asked, "What do you want to do now?"

"I'll go back and help you," she answered.

She became the best assistant I ever had. She boiled my three precious syringes in a little pot after each use, washed bandages and hung them in the sun to dry, swept the clinic's floors, helped with meals and even held patients down when we had to make an incision in surgery. From translator to nurse to cook, there was nothing she did not do.

And then one morning I woke up and she was gone. Apparently sometime during the night she had slipped away without leaving a note or saying goodbye. I was both mystified and disappointed. Several days later, though, I figured out the explanation. Exactly three weeks had passed since we had taken her little boy to the hospital in Lublin. I had been too involved in the daily work to keep track, but she had counted each day.

A week later I woke up after a night under the stars and found a handkerchief on the ground next to my head. It was filled with soil. Figuring it was one of those superstitious things that happened all the time, I put it on one of the clinic's shelves and thought nothing more about it until one of the local women urged me to untie the knots and look inside. Sure enough, along with the dirt, I found a note made out to the "Pani Doctor" that said, "From Mrs. W., whose last of thirteen children you have saved, blessed Polish soil."

Ah, so the boy lived.

A big smile landed on my face.

Then I glanced down at the note's final line. It said, "Blessed Polish soil." Just like that I understood everything. After getting up in the middle of the night, this woman had walked the twenty miles back to the hospital and picked up her son very much alive. From Lublin, she returned him to her own village, dug a handful of soil from her home and found a priest to bless it. Since the Nazis had exterminated most of the priests, I am sure that she had to look far and wide for one. But now her dirt was special, blessed by God. After delivering her gift to me, she went back home. Once I realized all this, that little bag of dirt became the most precious gift I had ever received.

And though I had no way of knowing, soon it would also save my life.

CHAPTER TEN

Butterflies

I talk about love and compassion, but my greatest lessons concerning the meaning of life came from visiting a site where the worst atrocities against humanity took place.

Before leaving Poland, I attended a ceremony for the opening of the schoolhouse we built. Then I traveled to Maidanek, one of Hitler's notorious death factories. Something compelled me to see one of these concentration camps with my own eyes. It was as if seeing would help me understand.

I knew of Maidanek's reputation. It was where my Polish friend lost her husband and twelve of her thirteen children. Yes, I knew it well.

But actually going there was something else.

The gates to this massive place were smashed open, but signs of its ominous past, where more than 300,000 people died, were still on chilling display. I noticed barbed wire, guard towers and the many rows of barracks where men, women, children and entire families spent their last days and hours. There were also several train cars. I looked inside. The sight was ghastly. Some contained women's hair intended for shipment back to Germany, where it would be turned into winter clothes. Others held glasses, jewelry, wedding rings and trinkets people carried for sentimental reasons. The last car I looked in was loaded with children's clothes, baby shoes and toys.

I climbed back down and shuddered. Could life be that cruel?

The stench of the gas chambers, and of death, that

unmistakable smell, hanging in the air, provided the answer.

But why?

How was it possible?

It was inconceivable to me. I walked around in the camp-grounds in disbelief. I asked, "How can men and women do such things to each other?" Then I got to the barracks. "How did people, especially mothers and children, survive those weeks and days before their certain deaths?" Inside I saw bare wooden bunks crammed together five deep. On the walls, people had carved their names, initials and drawings. What implements had they used? Rocks? Their fingernails? I looked more closely and noticed that one image was repeated over and over again.

Butterflies.

They were everywhere I looked. Some were crude. Others were quite detailed. I could not imagine butterflies in horrible places like Maidanek, Buchenwald or Dachau. However, the barracks were full of them. Each barracks I entered. Butterflies. "Why?" I asked myself. "Why butterflies?"

Surely they had some special meaning. What? For the next twenty-five years, I asked that question and hated myself for not having an answer.

I walked back outside, feeling the impact Maidanek was having on me. Yet I was not aware that being there was preparing me for my life's work. Then I just wanted to understand how human beings could act so murderously toward other humans, especially innocent children.

Then the quiet of my thoughts was interrupted. I heard the clear, calm and assured voice of a young woman responding to me. Her name was Golda.

"You would be capable of doing that too," she said.

I wanted to object, but I was so stunned that nothing came out of my mouth. "If you had been raised in Nazi Germany," she added.

I wanted to shout my disagreement. "Not me!" I was a pacifist. I had grown up in a nice family and in a peaceful country. I had never known poverty, hunger or discrimination. Golda read all this in my eyes and knowingly replied, "You would be surprised what you're capable of doing. If you had been raised in Nazi Germany you could have easily turned into the kind of person who would do that. There is a Hitler in all of us."

I wanted to understand, not argue, and since it was lunchtime I invited Golda to share my sandwich. She was strikingly beautiful and looked about my age. In another setting, we could easily have been friends, schoolmates or co-workers. As we ate, Golda told me how she came to hold such an opinion.

Born in Germany, Golda had been twelve when the Gestapo showed up at her father's business and took him away. She never saw him again. Then right after the war broke out, she and the rest of her family, including her grandparents, had been deported to Maidanek. One day the guards ordered them into the line they had watched so many step into and never return from. She and her family were among those who were stripped and pushed into the gas chamber. They screamed, begged, cried, prayed. But they had no chance or hope for dignity or survival as they were pushed to deaths worse than those of any cattle in a slaughterhouse.

Golda, this gorgeous young girl, had been the last person they tried to squeeze in before closing the door and turning on the gas. By some miracle, by some divine intervention, the door would not close with her in there. It was too crowded. In order to fill their daily quota, they simply yanked her out and pushed her into the fresh air. Since she was already on the death list, they presumed she was dead and no one ever called her name again. Thanks to an unusual oversight, her life was spared.

She had little time to grieve. Most of her energy was consumed by the basic task of staying alive. She scrambled to survive the Polish winter, find enough food and avoid diseases like typhoid or even a simple cold, which would prevent her from digging ditches or shoveling snow and would send her back to the gas chambers. To keep her spirits up, she imagined the camp being liberated. God had chosen her, she reasoned, to survive and tell future generations about the barbarity she had witnessed.

This was enough, she said, to keep her going through the harshest cold of winter. If she felt her energy fail, Golda closed her eyes and imagined the screams of her girlfriends who had been used as guinea pigs in experiments conducted by camp doctors, abused by camp guards or often both, and then she told herself, "I must live to tell the world. I must live to tell them the horrors these people committed." And Golda nourished this hate and determination to stay alive until the Allied forces arrived.

Then, when the camp was liberated and the gates opened, Golda was paralyzed by the rage and bitterness that gripped her. She did not see herself spending the rest of her valuable life spewing hatred. "Like Hitler," she said. "If I used my life, which was spared, to sow the seeds of hatred, I would not be any different than him. I would just be another victim trying to spread more and more hate. The only way we can find peace is to let the past be the past," she said.

In her own way she was answering all the questions that had popped into my head by being at Maidanek. Till then, I had not truly been aware of man's potential for savagery. But you only had to see the trainload of baby shoes or breathe the foul odor of death that lingered in the air like a ghostly pall to realize the inhumanity man was capable of. But then how do you explain Golda, someone who had experienced such cruelty and had instead chosen to forgive and love?

She explained that herself by saying, "If I can change one person's life from hatred and revenge to love and compassion, then I deserved to survive."

I understood and left Maidanek changed forever. I felt as if my life had started all over again.

I still wanted to attend medical school. But I decided the purpose of my life would be to ensure that future generations would not create another Hitler.

Of course, first I had to get back home.

Getting back to Switzerland was as perilous as anything else that I had done in the preceding months. Rather than go straight back, I decided to see a bit of Russia. I traveled by myself. With no money or visa, I packed my blanket, the few clothes I had and my bundle of Polish dirt into my backpack and set out on the road to Bialystok. By nightfall, I had crossed miles of isolated countryside without any sign of the dreaded Russian Army—my only concern—and so I prepared to camp out on a grassy hill. I had never felt so alone before, like a dot on the planet staring up at the billions of stars.

But it was momentary. Before I unfurled my blanket, I was approached by an old woman in a colorful, multilayered dress who seemed to appear from out of nowhere. Something about all the scarves and jewelry she wore seemed out of place. Then again, this was the Russian countryside, a dark, mystical place full of secrets. Speaking Russian, which I barely understood, she offered to read some cards for me, apparently looking for money. Uninterested in the fantasies she would no doubt tell me, I used bits of Polish, Russian and hand gestures to say that what I really needed was human company and a safe place to spend the night. Could she help?

Smiling, she gave the only answer possible—"the Gypsy camp."

It was a remarkable four days of singing, dancing and companionship. Before I set off again, I taught them a Swiss folk song. They played it as a farewell as I hitched my backpack up once more and walked down the road leading into Poland. I became misty-eyed that total strangers meeting in the middle of the night, people who had no language in common other than love and music in their hearts, could share so deeply and feel like brothers and sisters in such a brief time. I left feeling hopeful the world could mend itself after the war.

In Warsaw, the Quakers arranged a seat for me on a U.S. warplane carrying VIPs to Berlin. From there, I planned to catch a train to Zurich. I cabled my family to let them know when I would arrive home. "In time for dinner," I wrote, excitedly anticipating one of my mother's tasty meals and a good night's sleep in my own soft bed.

But the danger heightened in Berlin. Russian troops refused to let anyone without proper credentials cross from their side of the city—later to become part of East Germany—into the British-occupied sector in the west. At night, people disappeared off the streets, hoping to escape, at least temporarily, the fear and tension that was so palpable. Aided by strangers, I made it to a border checkpoint, where I stood for hours while growing tired, hungry and sick to my stomach. When it was apparent I could not make it across by myself, I persuaded a British officer who was driving a truck to hide me in a two-by-three-foot wooden crate and smuggle me into a safe zone near Hildesheim.

For the next eight hours I curled in a fetal position, concentrating on the emphatic warning he gave just before nailing the top shut: "*Please,* don't make a sound. Not a cough. Not a loud breath. Nothing until I remove the lid again." At each stop, I held my breath, fearful that if I moved even a finger it would be my last. I remember the light blinding me when the top was finally removed. I had never seen such bright light. The relief and gratitude I felt once I saw the British officer's face was matched only by the waves of nausea and weakness that swept through my body after he helped me out of my hiding place.

After declining his kind offer to share a good meal in an officers' mess, I started hiking toward home. At night, I unrolled my blanket in a cemetery and woke the next morning even sicker than before. I had no food or medicine. In my backpack, I found my bundle of Polish soil—the only thing besides my blanket that had not been stolen—and I knew that somehow I would make it.

I managed to lift my body, which pulsed with excruciating pain, and limp down the unpaved gravel road. Somehow I lasted for several hours. Finally, I collapsed in a meadow on the outskirts of a thick forest. I knew that I was very ill, but there was nothing to do but pray. I was starving and sweating with fever; my mind clouded over. In my delirium, I saw a montage of recent experiences like the clinic in Lucima, the butterflies in Maidanek and the girl Golda.

Ah, Golda. So precious. So strong.

Once I opened my eyes and imagined a small girl eating a sandwich as she rode by on a bicycle. My stomach twitched from hunger. For a moment, I contemplated stealing that sandwich right out of the little girl's hands. Whether she was real or not, I do not know. But at the moment I had the thought, I heard Golda's words: "There is a Hitler in all of us." Now I understood. It just depends on the circumstances.

In this case, they were on my side. A poor old woman found me sleeping while she was out collecting firewood. Somehow she carted me to a German hospital near Hildesheim. For several days, I drifted in and out of consciousness. During a period of clarity, I heard talk about an epidemic of typhoid that was killing scores of women. Figuring I was among that ill-fated lot, I asked for pencil and paper in order to write my family in case I never saw them again.

But I was too weak to hold the pencil. I asked my roommate and the nurse for help, but both refused. The bigots thought I was Polish. It was the same kind of prejudice I'd witness forty years later with AIDS patients. "Let the Polish pig die," they said disgustedly.

Such prejudice nearly killed me. Later that night I suffered a cardiac spasm and no one wanted to help the "Polish" girl. My poor body, withered to a frightening seventy-five pounds, had no fight left in it. Doubled over in bed, I faded fast. Fortunately, the doctor on duty that night took his oath seriously. Before it was too late, he administered an injection of strophanthin. By morning, I felt more like myself than I had since departing from Lucima. The color had returned to my cheeks. I sat up and ate breakfast. On his way out, the doctor asked, "How's my little Swiss girl today?" Swiss! As soon as the nurses and my roommate heard I was Swiss and not Polish, their attitudes toward me changed. Suddenly, they couldn't do enough to help.

The hell with them. Several weeks later, after much-needed rest and nourishment, I checked out. But before leaving, I told my prejudiced roommate and the nurses the story behind the Polish soil I kept in my rucksack. "Do you understand?" I explained. "There is no difference between the mother of a Polish child and the mother of a German child!"

The train ride back to Zurich gave me time to ponder the incredible education that I had received over the past eight months. I was definitely returning home wiser and more worldly. As the train rumbled down the tracks, I already heard myself telling my family everything—about the butterflies and the Polish-Jewish girl who taught me about the Hitler in all of us; about the Russian Gypsies who taught me about love and brotherhood that transcends language and nationality; about strangers like the poor woman who went out to gather firewood and got me to the hospital in time to survive.

Soon enough, I was back at the dinner table with my mother and father, sharing all the horrors I had seen . . . and all the many more reasons we had to be hopeful.

PART II

"The Bear"

CHAPTER ELEVEN

Home for Dinner

Thank goodness for bosses like Professor Amsler. He was a brilliant ophthalmologic surgeon, but that skill was outshone by the traits that made him a great human being, compassion and understanding. Less than a year after I had started my job at the University Hospital he had allowed me leave to do volunteer work, and then he welcomed me back into my old position when I showed up again. "It must be winter, because the little swallow flies back home," he said upon my return.

My old basement lab seemed like heaven. I resumed the same routine and research. But soon Professor Amsler recognized that I had changed and could handle more responsibility. He reassigned me to the children's ward, where I tested children who were losing their eyesight from sympathetic ophthalmia or a malignancy. My approach was different from that of their parents and doctors. I talked directly to the children, listened to their fears about going blind and noticed how candidly they responded. Again, I was acquiring the skills I would use later on.

I loved the work I did in my cellar lab with these sight-affected patients. The work took hours. There were lots of measurements and tests. It required our spending long periods together in darkness, perfect for conversation. Even the most reserved, cautious and shy patients opened up to me in that intimate setting. I was just a twenty-three-year-old lab tech, but I learned to listen like an older, more experienced psychiatrist.

Everything I did emphasized how much I wanted to become a

89

physician. I looked forward to passing the Matura, the university's difficult entrance exam, and made preliminary plans to take night school classes to fill in the gaps in my education, subjects like German, French and English literature, geometry and trigonometry and the most dreaded of all, Latin.

But then summer arrived, and news from the IVSP blew in on a warm breeze. A crew of volunteers was building an access road to a hospital in Recco, Italy. They desperately needed a cook. They did not even have to ask if I was interested, because several days later I was swinging a pick by day and singing around a campfire at night on the Italian Riviera. Nothing was more satisfying. My sweet Professor Amsler had guaranteed my job, and my parents had given their approval. By now they were all used to me.

There was just one rule. Before I left, my father had prohibited me from traveling behind the Iron Curtain. It was not safe, and he feared that I would vanish.

"If you go across the Iron Curtain, you are no longer my daughter," he said, trying to deter me by issuing the strongest possible punishment.

"Yes, sir," I replied.

Such silliness, I thought. Why would he worry like that when I was spending the summer in Italy?

For good reason. As work on the road sped to an early finish, the IVSP contacted me with an urgent request to reunite two children with their parents in Poland. Their mother was Swiss and their new stepfather was Polish, and they couldn't get out of the country. My previous work there made me the best candidate for this assignment. I spoke the language, knew my way around and didn't look suspicious. I had just hitchhiked through all the major Italian cities to see the incredible art. One more adventure before summer ended was fine with me. And a chance to see Poland once more. This was a gift from heaven.

The children, a boy, age eight, and a girl, age six, waited for me in Zurich. Before picking them up, I stopped at home to freshen up and pack new clothes. If my mother had been there, I might have averted later problems. But the apartment was empty. Forgetting my father's admonition, I scribbled a brief greeting and described my plans.

At the train station, the chief of the IVSP's Zurich office added one more task to my mission of mercy. He asked if I would check out the conditions at an orphanage in Prague, Czechoslovakia. Despite the risk, I agreed. And any concern about the danger faded during an uneventful trip to Warsaw, where, despite the Communist rule, I dropped off my charges and then poked around the city overnight. I was pleasantly surprised to see smiling faces, flowers in marketplaces and much more food than I'd found there two years earlier.

Prague presented an extremely different picture. Just passing through the barriers outside the city required a dehumanizing strip search at the checkpoint as if I were a criminal. The disgusting guards even stole my umbrella and some other belongings. It was the first time during all my travels that I had been frightened. As for the city, I remember a pall of negativity and mistrust everyplace I went. Empty shops, grim faces, not a flower in sight. All the spirit had been suffocated.

The orphanage turned out to be a nightmare. My heart broke for the children who lived there. It was disgusting. Not clean, not enough food and, worst of all, no love. However, there was nothing I could do about it. Police agents monitored me closely and eventually told me to my face that I was not welcome there.

Although furious, I wasn't stupid. There was no way I could fight the powerful Czech Army and win. But I wasn't running away defeated either. Before leaving the orphanage, I emptied out my backpack and gave away my clothes, shoes, blankets and whatever else I carried. On the short trip back to Zurich, I wished I could've done more in Prague but settled for the glimmer of hope that remained in Warsaw.

"Jejdje Polsak nie ginewa," I sang softly. "Poland is not yet lost. No, Poland is not yet lost."

Like all children, I got excited every time I returned home from a trip, particularly this one. Outside the apartment door, which couldn't contain the rich aroma of my mother's delicious cooking, I heard a lively discussion taking place amid the clatter of dinner dishes. The loudest voice, which I hadn't heard for a long time, made my heart leap with excitement—it was my brother's. Ernst had been living in Pakistan and India for years.

Our contact had been through letters and superficial at that, making this rare visit extra special. Now we'd have plenty of time to catch up and be a whole family as in the old days.

But that turned out to be wishful thinking. While I paused on the stoop to dream about what Ernst looked like after so much time, the front door suddenly opened. My father, who had spotted me through the window, stood in the doorway, blocking me from entering. He was angry. "Who are you?" he asked sternly. "We don't know you."

I expected my father to grin and say he was joking, but the door slammed shut and I knew he must have found out where I'd gone. I didn't remember the note I'd hastily scribbled, but I sensed that he was punishing me for being disobedient. I heard his footsteps across the wooden floor. Then silence. The conversation resumed inside, albeit less spirited than before, and neither my mother nor my sisters rescued me. Knowing my father, he probably forbade them to go to the door.

If this was the price I paid for doing what felt right rather than what was expected, then I had no choice other than to be as tough as or tougher than my father. After some anguished moments, I finally wandered down the Klosbachstrasse, ending up in the little coffee shop at the trolley station, where there was a bathroom and something to eat. I figured I would sleep in my lab, only I didn't have any clothes. I'd given away everything I had in Prague.

I stepped into a coffee shop and ordered something to eat. I had no doubt that my mother was upset at my father but powerless to change him. My sisters would have certainly helped, but they had lives of their own. Erika was married, and Eva was engaged to Seppli Bucher, a champion skier and poet. I was definitely on my own, and it was a mess. But I had no regrets. Appropriately enough, I remembered a poem that my grandmother had hanging over the guest bed, where I had spent many nights as a child. Roughly translated, it said:

> *Always when you think*
> *you cannot make it anymore*
> *from out of nowhere*
> *comes a little light.*

This little light
will renew your strength
and give you the energy
to go one more step.

I was so tired I started to fall asleep at the table. Suddenly I was startled awake by someone calling my name. When I looked up, I saw my friend Cilly Hofmeyr. She waved from across the coffee shop and then sat down at my table. Cilly had graduated from Canton Hospital as a promising speech therapist at the same time I qualified as a lab technician. We hadn't seen each other since then, but Cilly was as outgoing and personable as I remembered. Soon she was telling me how badly she wanted to move out of her mother's house. "I want to be more independent," she said.

It turned out Cilly had spent weeks searching for an apartment, but found only one affordable place. It was an attic apartment, ninety-seven steps up, no elevator, though it had breathtaking views of the Lake of Zurich, plus running water and easy access to public transportation. The only catch was that the landlord would only rent the apartment to a tenant who also agreed to take the one-room cubby across the hall.

She was disappointed. I thought it sounded perfect.

"Let's take it," I shouted before I had even explained my predicament.

The next day we signed the lease and moved in. My furniture, except for a great big antique desk, came from the Salvation Army, while Cilly, a talented musician, somehow got a baby grand piano into her place. Later that afternoon I sneaked back home and told my mother where I was living, including the view I had from my small window. I also picked up some clothes and invited her and my sisters to visit.

Although my drapes were actually old bedsheets, my new home was a cozy nest. Cilly and I entertained almost every night. Her friends from the local chamber orchestra provided wonderful music and my collection of homesick foreign students from the university added intellectual conversation. One Turkish architectural student brought his own brass coffeepot and halva for dessert. My sisters visited frequently. It was not a great place, not my parents' home, but I would not have traded it for anything.

93

In the fall of 1950, I focused on getting into medical school. For the next year I put in my hours at the lab with Professor Amsler and then spent the night studying for the Matura. The course-work ranged from trigonometry and Shakespeare to geography and physics. Ordinarily it took three years to prepare, but I worked at my own accelerated pace and was ready in just twelve months.

At the appropriate time, I filled out the application but I did not have the 500 Swiss francs for the entrance fee. My mother could not help; she would have had to ask my father for that amount of money. For a moment, my situation looked hopeless. But then my sister Erika and her husband, Ernst, loaned me the money that they had saved for a new kitchen. It was 500 francs.

I took the Matura in early September 1951. It was five straight days of intensive tests, including essays. In order to pass, your combined results had to be above a certain average. I whizzed through physics, math, biology, zoology and botany. Latin was a catastrophe. I had done so well in everything else that the old professor administering the exam was brokenhearted when he had to give me a failing grade. Fortunately I had planned on that when strategizing the combined average of my scores. I had no doubt that I passed.

The official notification that I passed came in the mail on the day before my father's birthday. Although we still had not spoken, I made him a special birthday present, a calendar on which I wrote, in the relevant dates, "Happy Birthday" and "Passed the Matura." I dropped it off at home that afternoon and then waited outside his office the next morning for his reaction. I knew he would be proud.

My hunch was right. Although at first my father didn't look pleased to see me, his grimace changed to a smile. It wasn't exactly an apology, but it was the first hint of affection I'd gotten from him in more than a year. That was okay. The ice continued to melt. After I returned from the lab that night, my sisters showed up at my apartment with a message from him: "Father wants you to come home for dinner."

Over a wonderful meal, he toasted my achievement. But all of us were there again, and we celebrated much more than my test results.

CHAPTER TWELVE

Medical School

In my work on death and dying, I was influenced by C. G. Jung more than any other psychiatrist. As a first-year medical student I often saw the legendary Swiss psychiatrist taking long walks through Zurich. He was a familiar sight on sidewalks and around the lake, always appearing lost in deep thought. I felt an eerie connection to him, a familiarity that told me we would have hit it off magically.

Sadly, though, I never introduced myself, and in fact went out of my way to avoid the great man. As soon as I spotted Jung, I either crossed the street or changed my direction. Now I regret it. But back then I thought that if I spoke to him I would become a psychiatrist and that was at the very bottom of my list.

From the moment I enrolled in medical school, I planned on becoming a country doctor. In Switzerland, that is expected, part of the deal. After graduating, the new doctors take over a country practice. It is like an apprenticeship, introducing new doctors to general medicine before they search for a specialty, like surgery or orthopedic medicine. If they are so inclined, they stay put in a country practice, which was what I foresaw myself doing. But that was seven years into the future.

It was a good system, though. It turned out good doctors whose first consideration was the patient, then payment.

I got off to a good start in medical school, flying through the basic natural sciences, chemistry and biochemistry and physiology. But my introduction to anatomy nearly got me kicked out of school. On the first day, everyone around me spoke a foreign language. Thinking I was in the wrong classroom, I got up to leave. The professor, a rude disciplinarian, stopped his lecture and upbraided me for interrupting him, even though I tried to explain. "You aren't confused," he said. "Women should be at home cooking and sewing rather than studying medicine."

I was mortified. Later I realized that one-third of the class were from Israel, part of an arrangement between the two governments, and that the foreign language I heard was Hebrew. Then I had another run-in with the same anatomy professor. Upon hearing that several of the first-year students, including me, were trying to raise money for a destitute student, one of the Israelis, rather than studying, he expelled the student who organized the charitable effort and then told me to "go home and become a seamstress instead."

These were tough lessons, but I thought this professor had forgotten a basic one, and I risked my future career to tell him so. "We were just trying to help a fellow human being in distress," I said. "Didn't you take an oath to do the same thing when you became a doctor?"

My point was well taken. The student who had been expelled was reinstated and I continued to help others, usually one of the foreign students. I befriended some Indian students. One had a friend who had been partially blinded after a rat bit him in the eye. He was hospitalized in Professor Amsler's department, where I continued to work five nights a week. The student, from a village near the Himalayas, was scared and depressed and hadn't eaten for days.

From personal experience, I knew how terrible it was to be sick far from home. So I arranged for some familiar curry-flavored Indian food to be served to him. I also got permission for one of his Indian friends to stay in his room during nonvisiting hours as he got ready for surgery. Little touches. But his strength quickly returned.

In appreciation, I received an invitation from Indian Prime Minister Nehru to an official reception at the Indian consulate in Bern. It was a fancy event held in the outdoor garden. I wore a beautiful sari donated by my Indian friends. Nehru's daughter, Indira Gandhi, the country's future prime minister, presented me

96

with flowers and a citation, though her personal kindness meant much more to me. During the reception, she saw me ask her father to sign a copy of his famous book *The Unity of India.* "Not now," he barked. Embarrassed and hurt, I jumped back and literally landed in her outstretched arms. "Don't be scared," she said soothingly. "I will have him sign it."

Sure enough, two minutes later she handed him my book. He signed it and handed it back, smiling as if nothing had ever happened. Years later, I was asked to sign thousands of books, once even while sitting on the toilet at John F. Kennedy International Airport in New York. As much as I wanted to shout, "Not now," I refrained from embarrassing myself and startling the other person who'd bought my book, remembering instead the lesson I'd learned from the Indian prime minister.

School was consuming without being burdensome. Maybe I was more accustomed to heavier workloads than most people. Or better organized. My nights were spent in the ophthalmology lab, which gave me a regular income. Not that I needed much to live on. Most times I took a sandwich with me for dinner, but on occasion I joined classmates in the student cafeteria. I don't remember having much time to study except in the mornings when I took the trolley to school.

Fortunately I had a photographic memory when it came to recalling classwork and lectures. But the downside to that was boredom, particularly in anatomy. During one review lecture, a girlfriend of mine and I sat high up in the amphitheater, gossiping about our lives, past and future. For fun, she scanned the large room and then pointed at a handsome Swiss medical student. "That's him," she said laughingly. "That's my future husband."

We laughed. "Now you pick your husband," she said.

I looked around. There was a group of American students directly across the room from us. They had a reputation for obnoxious behavior. They joked constantly and whispered comments that other students found offensive about the cadavers. I hated them. Despite that, my eyes landed on one of them, a good-looking, dark-haired guy. Somehow I had never noticed him before. Nor did I know his name. "Him," I said. "He's the one for me."

More laughter at our girlish impulsiveness.

Deep down, though, neither of us doubted that we'd eventually marry those men. It was left up to time and "coincidence."

As far as I was concerned, nothing went right for me when it concerned anatomy class. It started off bad and then appeared to get worse when we moved from basic coursework into the pathology lab, where students were grouped in fours and assigned to a single cadaver. I swore the professor was trying to get even with me for our past disagreements when I saw whom he'd placed me with—three of the Americans, including the handsome young man I'd chosen as my future husband.

My first impression of them as a group, based on how they handled the corpse, was not a good one. They made jokes about the dead man's body, jumped rope with his intestines and teased me about the size of his testicles. It wasn't funny. I thought they were disrespectful, insensitive cowboys. And although it wasn't a particularly romantic or cute way to meet a future beau, I did not keep my opinion a secret. Such derogatory behavior and joking, I said sternly, were grounds for expulsion. It also distracted me from learning all the blood vessels, nerves and muscles.

They listened politely, but only one of them reacted—my American. At the peak of my explosion, he offered an apologetic smile and extended his hand. "Hi," he said, "my name is Ross—Emanuel Ross."

I was immediately disarmed. Emanuel Ross. He was broad-shouldered, athletic and much bigger than I was. And he was from New York. You could hear that in his voice. It sounded "Brooklyn" before you even asked where he was from. Then he added one more thing: "Friends call me Manny."

Even after we became lab partners, it took three months before Manny asked me out for a movie and a bite to eat at a café. I knew he had a lot of good-looking girlfriends, but we developed an easy friendship that allowed us to be open with each other. Manny, the youngest of three children, had an unusually tough childhood. Both of his parents were deaf-mutes. His father died when Manny was six; the family moved into his uncle's small apartment. They were very poor. The only gift he ever received from his father, a stuffed tiger, was taken, and then lost, by hospital nurses when he had his tonsils out at five. Though many years had passed, I saw that the loss still pained Manny. To console him, I told him about my rabbit, Blackie.

Manny, I also learned, had worked his way through school, served in the Navy and graduated pre-med from NYU. To avoid the glut of ex-GIs vying for spots in overcrowded U.S. medical schools, he chose the University of Zurich, even though it meant wrestling with lectures in German and classroom discussions in Schweizerdeutsch. Manny, who ascribed some of his success to my help as a translator, was the first young man I dated who made me think of the future. Before summer vacation, I taught Manny to ski. When we returned for our second year, I started plotting how to get rid of his other female admirers.

During the second year, we were introduced to actual patients. I had a detective's flair for making the proper diagnosis quickly and a fondness for pediatrics that I supposed had something to do with my having been critically ill as a child. Or it might've been related to memories I had of my sister Erika hospitalized there. Fortunately, I didn't waste much energy on that question, since I was wrapped up in figuring out a potentially bigger problem—introducing Manny to my family without my father pitching a fit. The coming holidays gave me a chance.

Ordinarily, Christmas was a special day reserved just for family, but the week before I got my mother's okay to invite three handpicked American classmates, including Manny, to her famous Christmas dinner. I'd given a real sob story, which was basically true, about how these students were far from home, lonely and unable to afford a good holiday dinner, embellishing just enough so that my mother spent days preparing all sorts of traditional Swiss treats to impress the Americans. Meanwhile, we gently prepared my father for the fact that this year's Christmas would be more than just family.

On the big night, Manny instantly thrilled my mother by bringing fresh flowers and all three guys won her everlasting favor by clearing the table and washing the dishes, something Swiss men didn't ever do on their own. My father served some excellent wine and brandy, and that naturally led to a jovial sing-along around the piano lasting till the dozens of candles that filled the living room with a warm glow burned way down. Around ten o'clock, I gave a prearranged signal for my friends to go. "Pretty soon it will be eleven," I announced none too subtly. If guests overstayed their welcome, my father let them know by opening the front door and all the windows, even if it was ten degrees below zero outside, and I wanted to avoid that.

But my father truly enjoyed himself. "They're very nice guys," he said afterward. "And Manny is the nicest of all. He's the best young man you've ever brought to the house." True, he had fit in. However, there was still one important fact about Manny that my father didn't know, though this buoyant moment provided the perfect chance to drop that bombshell. "And just think, he's a Jew," I said. Silence. Before my father, who I knew had no fondness for Zurich's Jewish community, could respond, I ran off to help my mother in the kitchen, expecting to have to defend my friend sooner or later.

Thankfully, it wasn't that night. My father went directly to bed without comment, saving his thoughts till morning. Over breakfast, he dropped a bombshell of his own. "You can bring Manny to our home anytime you like," he said. Within a few months, I didn't even have to invite Manny. Accepted as one of the family, he occasionally came for dinner even if I wasn't there.

As expected, there was a wedding in 1955. No, not mine, even though Manny and I had grown close enough to understand that we'd eventually marry. Just not before finishing school. The bride and groom were my sister Eva and her fiancé, Seppli, who pledged their eternal love in the tiny chapel where my family had worshipped for generations. Ever since they'd become a serious couple, my parents hinted that Seppli might not be the greatest catch for my sister. A doctor? A lawyer? Yes. A businessman, certainly. A skier/poet? That was a problem.

Not to me. I defended Seppli up and down. He was a bright, sensitive, gentle soul who appreciated the mountains, flowers and sunshine as much as I did. During weekends the three of us spent at our mountain cabin in Amden, Seppli always had a broad smile when he skied, sang, yodeled or played the guitar and violin. On the few times Manny joined all of us there, I noticed that he tolerated sleeping on a mattress without bedding and cooking on a wood stove, and he looked impressed when I pointed out the different fauna and sights in the forests, but he was always relieved to get back to the city.

The next year didn't allow for any mountain retreats. Although it was the last of my seven years in medical school, it was the hardest. In the Swiss equivalent of an internship, I began the year by taking over a general medical practice in Niederweningen for a nice young doctor who was attending military service for three weeks. Having come from a modern teaching hospital, I suffered a blast of culture shock as he hastily guided me through his home office, showing me the lab, the X-ray equipment and an idiosyncratic filing system containing the names of patients from seven local farming villages.

"Seven villages?" I questioned.

"Yes, so you'll have to learn to ride a motorcycle," he said.

We never discussed the when part of that. A few hours after he left, I received my first emergency call. It was in one of the outlying villages, about fifteen minutes away. I strapped my black medical bag on the back of the motorcyle, kick-started it as I had been shown and took off on my first motorcycle ride ever. I didn't even have a driver's license.

I started out okay. But about one-third of the way up the hill, I heard my medical bag slip off the back. Then there was a loud crash. All my medical equipment hit the ground and scattered. As soon as I turned around to look at the mess, I knew I had made a big mistake. The bike hit a pothole, took a path of its own, spun out of control and dropped me off in a spot roughly between the bag and where the motorcycle eventually stopped.

Such was my introduction to a country practice, and also the town's introduction to me. Unbeknownst to me, the whole town had watched out their windows. Everybody knew there was a new woman doctor, and as soon as they heard my motorcycle put-putting up the hill, they ran to see what I looked like. After I picked myself up, I looked scraped and bloody in a few places. Some men helped straighten out the bike. And eventually I made it to the right house, where I took care of an old man who was having a heart scare. I think he felt better as soon as he saw that I looked worse than he did.

After three weeks in the wilds, treating everything from scraped knees to cancer patients, I returned to my classes exhausted but more

101

confident. Even though I wasn't interested in my two remaining classes, I had no problem with either obstetrics/gynecology or cardiology. Ahead were the State Board exams, six months of tedium and pressure that needed to be conquered in order to become a doctor. And after that? Manny pushed for us to go to America after school, while I felt an urge to do volunteer work in India. Clearly we had our differences, but I trusted my instincts that the good outweighed the bad.

It was a difficult time, and then something happened that made it even harder.

CHAPTER THIRTEEN

Good Medicine

The Boards were daylong oral and written interrogations that covered everything we had learned over the past seven years. They examined both character and clinical knowledge. I passed without difficulty, worrying more about how Manny was going to do than about my own score.

But there were things doctors faced that were not taught in medical school, and I faced just such a test in the midst of taking my final exams. It started at Eva and Seppli's apartment. I had stopped for coffee and pastries, needing a distraction from the pressure of taking tests. But as we talked, I noticed Seppli looked pale and tired, definitely not his usual upbeat self, and thinner than normal, prompting me to ask how he was feeling. "A little stomachache," he said. "My doctor says I have an ulcer."

Intuitively, I knew my brother-in-law, this strong, relaxed mountain man, didn't have an ulcer, and over the next few weeks I made a pest of myself, checking on his condition daily and then contacting his doctor, who had no patience for my second-guessing his diagnosis. "You medical students are all alike," he scoffed. "You think you know everything."

I believed that Seppli was seriously ill and I was not alone. Eva had similar fears. She watched and worried as her husband's health waned. She was greatly relieved to finally be able to talk about it, even after I raised the possibility of cancer. We took Seppli to the best doctor I knew, an old country practitioner (a part-time university professor), who actually "listened" to patients and had a reputation as a marvelous diagnostician. After a brief examination, he confirmed our worst suspicion and wasted no time scheduling surgery for the next week.

There had been hundreds of questions on my Boards, but not like the ones that were in my head. I took Seppli to the hospital; the surgeon had already invited me to assist during the operation. If the result was serious, I would call Eva and say, "I was right." The rest would be up to fate. And as for Seppli, just twenty-eight years old and married for less than a year, he handled this unfortunate twist of fate with the same grace he exhibited on the ski slopes.

I tried to do the same as we entered the operating room. It was hard to watch, but I never took my eyes off Seppli, even as the surgeon made the first incision. Once Seppli's stomach was open, it got even harder. First we saw a small ulcer along the inner wall. Then the surgeon shook his head. Seppli's stomach was full of a thick malignancy. There was nothing to do. "Sorry, but your hunch was right," the surgeon said.

My sister accepted the news with painful silence. "No, there was nothing to do for him," I explained, and then we shared a feeling of impotence and anger, particularly toward Seppli's first doctor, who never considered such a grave possibility when there might still have been time to save this young life.

While Seppli slept in the recovery room, I sat on his bed and pictured the beautiful old-fashioned horse-drawn carriage that had ferried him and Eva less than twelve months ago from our house to the traditional wedding chapel across town. Back then, the world had seemed in order. Both my sisters were married, everybody was terribly happy, and I expected to follow them down the aisle in the future. But looking at Seppli, I realized you couldn't depend on the future. Life was about the present.

Indeed, as Seppli awoke, he accepted his condition without asking any questions, listening to his doctor tell him exactly what he needed to know while I clasped his hand tightly as if my strength would help him. That was normal wishful thinking but not realistic. After several weeks, Seppli went home, where my sister provided him with care, comfort and love during the final months of his life.

On a gorgeous fall day in 1957 years of hard work finally paid off. "You have passed," said the university's chief examiner. "You are a physician."

My celebration was bittersweet. I was depressed because of Seppli, and I was also disappointed that a six-month surgical project in India had fallen through at the last moment. The bad news was so late in coming that I had already given away all my winter clothes. But if that had not happened, I probably would not have married Manny.

We loved each other, but we were not the perfect couple. For starters, he opposed my trip to India. After he finished his last semester, he saw us moving to America. I had a very low opinion of the United States, thanks to the obnoxious medical students I had met.

But when my plans changed I decided to gamble. I chose Manny and a future in the United States.

Ironically, my application for a visa was turned down by U.S. embassy officials. Brainwashed by McCarthyism, they assumed that anyone like me who traveled to Poland must be a Communist. But that point became irrelevant when Manny and I married in February 1958. We had a small civil ceremony, largely so Seppli could serve as best man before it was too late. The very next day he entered a hospital. As it turned out, he never would have made it till the larger, formal wedding we planned when Manny finished school in June.

Till then, I accepted a temporary position in Langenthal, where an adored country doctor had suddenly died, leaving his wife and son without any income or medical coverage. Most of the money I earned went to them, but I had whatever I needed and that was enough. Like the doctor who preceded me, I sent a bill out once and if someone wasn't able to pay I didn't worry about it. Almost all the patients gave something. If not money, then they showed up with baskets teeming with fruit and vegetables, even a handmade dress which fit me perfectly. On Mother's Day, I received so many flowers my office looked like a funeral parlor.

My saddest day in Langenthal was also my busiest. From the moment I opened the door in the morning, the waiting room was full. In the midst of stitching up a gash in a little girl's leg, I got a phone call from Seppli, whose voice barely rose above a whisper.

With a little girl half sutured and crying on the table, it was impossible to talk. Seppli made one request. Could I come see him? No, I explained unhappily, the waiting room was packed and I still had house calls. I'd already planned a trip to visit him. In two days. Trying to sound positive, I said, "I'll see you then."

Sadly, it didn't work out that way, which I'm sure was why Seppli called, urging me to see him one last time. Like most dying people who've accepted the inexorable transition from this world to the other side, he knew what precious little time remained to say goodbye. Sure enough, early the next morning Seppli died.

After Seppli's funeral, there were times in Langenthal when I walked through the rolling fields, breathing the fresh air sweetened by bursts of colorful spring flowers, while sensing Seppli was somewhere nearby. Often I talked to him until I felt better. Still, I never forgave myself for not having gone to see him.

I knew better than to ignore a dying patient's sense of urgency. Out in the country, health care was a shared experience. There was always a grandparent, parent, aunt, cousin, child or neighbor to help care for a sick patient. The same went for the very sick and the dying. Everyone pitched in—friends, family and neighbors. It was just understood that people did this for each other. In fact, my greatest satisfaction as a new physician came not at the clinic or while making house calls but from visiting patients who needed a friend, reassuring words or a few hours of companionship.

Medicine had its limits, a fact not taught in medical school. Another fact not taught there: a compassionate heart can heal almost anything. A few months in the country convinced me that being a good doctor had nothing to do with anatomy, surgery or prescribing the right medication. The biggest help a doctor could give a patient was to be a good, caring, sensitive, loving human being.

CHAPTER 14

Elisabeth Kübler-Ross, M.D.

෴

I was a grown woman, a practicing physician, and I was about to get married, but my mother treated me like a little girl. She got my hair done, took me to a makeup specialist and forced me to do all sorts of girly rubbish I could barely stand. She also told me not to complain about going to America, since Manny was an intelligent, handsome man who could marry any woman. "He probably wants you to help him during his final exams," she said.

It was a jab of insecurity on her part. She wanted me to count my blessings. But I already felt fortunate.

After Manny passed his Boards, without my assistance, we got married. It was a grand affair. My father was the only one who did not have a great time. Slowed by a broken hip he had suffered months earlier, he was not his normal graceful and princely self on the dance floor, and that depressed him. But he more than made up for it with his wedding present, a recording of him performing some of his favorite songs while my sister Eva accompanied him splendidly on the piano.

Afterward, my whole family went to the World's Fair in Brussels. Then they saw Manny and me, plus several of his friends who had attended the wedding, board the *Liberté*, the enormous cruise ship that was taking us to America. No amount of wonderful food, sun and dancing on the deck could alleviate the mixed feelings I had about leaving Switzerland for a country I had no interest in. Yet I let myself be drawn along without argument and from what I wrote in my journal I reasoned it was a journey I had to take.

> How do these geese know when to fly to the sun? Who tells them the seasons? How do we, humans, know when it is time to move on? How do we know when to go? As with the migrant birds, so surely with us, there is a voice within, if only we would listen to it, that tells us so certainly when to go forth into the unknown.

The night before arriving in the United States, I dreamed of myself dressed as an Indian on horseback riding across the desert. The sun in my dream was so hot I woke up with a parched throat. I was also suddenly thirsty for this new adventure. I told Manny that as a child I had drawn Indian shields and symbols and had danced on a flat rock like a warrior despite never having been exposed to American Indian culture. Was my dream an accident? Not likely. In a strange way, it calmed me. Like an inner voice, it gave me the sense that the unknown could actually be a home-coming.

It was for Manny. In a heavy downpour, he pointed out the Statue of Liberty to me. Thousands of people waited on the dock to greet the ship's passengers, including Manny's mother, who was deaf and mute, and his sister. For years, I had heard so much about them. Now I had just as many questions. What would they be like? Would they welcome a foreigner into the family? A non-Jew?

His mother was a doll whose joy at seeing her doctor son showed in her eyes as clearly as any sentence she might've spoken. His sister was another story. We were searching for our fifteen suitcases, crates and boxes when she found us. Manny got a big hug from this Long Island woman who had a ton of freshly coiffed gorgeous hair and new clothes. Then she studied my dripping hair and wet clothes as if I'd swum behind the boat and gave Manny a look that asked, "Is this the best you could do?"

After getting through customs, where my medical bag was confiscated, we went to Manny's sister-in-law's for dinner. She lived in Lynbrook, Long Island. At dinner, I unintentionally committed a sin by asking for a glass of milk. The irony was I never drank milk and would've preferred a brandy. But I thought everyone in America drank milk. Wasn't America "the land of milk and honey"? So I asked for one. Instead I got a sharp kick under the table from my husband. It was a kosher house, he explained.

"She'll have to learn about keeping kosher," my sister-in-law said snidely.

Later I entered the kitchen, hoping for a moment alone, and found my sister-in-law standing in front of the refrigerator, nibbling a piece of ham. Suddenly I was in a better mood. "I have no intention of keeping kosher," I said. "And I presume you are not totally kosher either."

My attitude improved somewhat when Manny and I moved into our own apartment several weeks later. The apartment was small but conveniently close to Glen Cove Community Hospital, where we both had rotating internships. Once work started—even though the schedule was grueling and the pay not enough to carry us through meals to the end of the month—I felt appreciably happier. There was something immensely comforting to me about wearing a white lab coat and having a roster of patients to occupy my thoughts and energy.

My days began early, when I fixed Manny breakfast, and then both of us worked late into the night. We returned home together, with barely enough strength to drag ourselves into bed. Every other weekend Manny and I were on duty, covering the 250-bed hospital by ourselves. We complemented each other's strengths. Manny was a meticulous, logical medical detective, excellent at pathology and histology. I was intuitive and calm, adept at making the snap decisions necessary in the emergency room.

We rarely had time for anything but work, and if we had extra time we did not have the money to do anything. There were exceptions. Once Manny's boss gave us two tickets to the Bolshoi Ballet, a special treat that excited us. We dressed in our fanciest clothes and took the train into Manhattan. But as soon as the lights went down I fell asleep and did not wake up until after the last curtain call.

Most of my difficulties had to do with adapting to a new culture. I remember one young man who had been admitted to the hospital emergency room with a serious ear problem. He was strapped to a stretcher, the usual procedure. But while he waited for an ENT specialist, he asked me if he could go to the rest room. Aware that the ENT specialist could come at any moment, I was not about to let him go anywhere and waste the doctor's time.

In addition, I had never heard the term "rest room" before. So before leaving on my rounds, I said, "You'll never get as much rest as you will by remaining right where you are."

On my next visit, a nurse was freeing him to go to the bathroom. I stood red-faced as she explained, "Doctor, his bladder was ready to rupture."

An even more humiliating moment occurred while I assisted in the operating room. During the routine procedure, the surgeon flirted shamelessly with the nurse, virtually ignoring me even though I handed him the instruments he needed. Suddenly, the patient started to bleed. The surgeon, snapping out of his infatuation with the nurse, yelled, "Shit!" Again, I was unfamiliar with this term. I looked over the instrument tray and then in a moment of panic said apologetically, "I don't know which one is shit."

Later on, Manny explained why everyone had laughed at me. But he was often as amused as everyone else by what he called my "banana skin episodes." The worst one occurred the night Manny's boss and his wife took us out for dinner to an elegant restaurant. For cocktails, I ordered a screwdriver, and when the main course was served the waiter asked if I wanted another drink. Trying for a joke, but unaware of what I was saying, I replied, "No, thanks. I've been screwed enough." The force of Manny's foot on my tibia told me I wasn't as humorous or clever as I intended.

I knew such mistakes were inevitable, part of adjusting to the United States. Nothing was as tough as not celebrating Christmas with my family. If not for the hospital librarian, a woman of Scandinavian descent, inviting us to her home for dinner, I might have run back to Switzerland before New Year's. She had a real Christmas tree, lit by actual candles as ours were back home, and as I wrote in a letter to my parents, "in the darkest night I found my little candle."

I thanked God for that night, but it didn't make me fit in any better than before. My Long Island neighbors were women who

110

gossiped over backyard fences about their analysts, comparing the most intimate matters as if nothing was private. And that wasn't the height of tastelessness, I was more offended by what I saw in the children's ward. Mothers, dressed up like fashion models on display, arrived with expensive toys that were supposed to show how much they cared about their sick children. The bigger the toy, the more they loved them, right? No wonder they all needed analysts.

One day in the children's ward I watched a spoiled brat throw a colossal fit when his mother forgot to bring a toy. Instead of saying, "Hi, Mom, thanks for visiting," he ranted, "Where's my gift?" and sent his panicked mother scurrying to the gift shop. I was appalled. What were these American mothers and their children thinking? Didn't they have any values? What good was all that stuff when what a sick child really needed was a parent to hold his hand and talk openly and honestly about life?

Because I was disgusted by these children and their parents, when it came time for interns to pick specialties Manny decided on a residency in pathology at Montefiore Hospital in the Bronx while I signed up to deal with what I called "the depraved minority"—pediatrics. Competition for the roughly two dozen residency slots with Columbia Presbyterian Medical Center's renowned Babies Hospital was intense, especially for foreigners. But Dr. Patrick O'Neil, the broad-minded veteran medical director who interviewed me, had never heard a reason like mine for wanting to go into pediatrics. "I can't stand those kids," I said. "Or their mothers."

Shocked and bemused, Dr. O'Neil nearly fell out of his chair. His look demanded further clarification. "If I could work with them, then I could understand them better," I explained. Then I added, "And hopefully tolerate them too."

Despite its unorthodoxy, the interview went well. At the end, Dr. O'Neil, looking for more than a simple yes-no answer, explained that the schedule, which required twenty-four-hour duty every other night, was too exhausting for pregnant residents. Aware of the information he wanted from me, I assured Dr. O'Neil that I had no plans to start a family yet. Two months later, I snatched a letter from Columbia Presbyterian from the mail, then hugged Manny, who was set to begin his residency in the summer. I was accepted—the first foreigner the prestigious hospital accepted for a pediatric residency.

Our celebration included the purchase of a new turquoise Chevy Impala, a splurge that allowed Manny to beam with pride. It was as if he saw a prosperous future in its shiny finish. This was followed by more good news. After several mornings of unpleasant nausea, I found out that I was pregnant. I always saw myself as a mother and therefore was thrilled. On the other hand, the pregnancy jeopardized my coveted residency. Hadn't Dr. O'Neil clearly explained the hospital's rule? No pregnant residents. Yes, it had been quite clear.

For a brief time, I toyed with the idea of not telling. It was June and I would not even show for another three or four months. By then, I would have three months of residency to my credit. I thought perhaps if Dr. O'Neil saw how hard I worked, he would make an exception. But I could not lie. Dr. O'Neil seemed genuinely disappointed to disqualify me, but there were no exceptions to the rule. The best he could do was promise to hold a spot open for me the next year.

That was nice, but it did not help the spot I was in at the moment. I needed a job. Manny's residency at Montefiore was going to pay $105 a month, not nearly enough to cover our expenses, never mind the addition of a baby. I did not know what to do. It was so late, every decent residency in the city would already be filled.

Then one night Manny told me he had just heard of an open residency position in the psychiatric ward at Manhattan State Hospital. I was not especially excited. Manhattan State Hospital was a mental institution, a public repository for the least desirable and most disturbed people. It was run by a crazy Swiss psychiatrist who drove his residents away. No one wanted to work for him. And to top it off, I hated psychiatry. It was last on my list of specialties.

But we needed to pay our rent and put food on the table. I also needed something to do.

So I interviewed with Dr. D. After chatting like neighbors in our native language, I left with the promise of a research fellowship and a salary of $400 per month. All of a sudden, we felt flush. Manny and I rented an adorable one-bedroom apartment on East Ninety-sixth Street in Manhattan. In the back, there was a little garden, which I fixed up one weekend for flowers and vegetables by carrying buckets of dirt in from Long Island. That night I ignored a slight bleeding. Then two days later I passed out in the operating room. I woke up as a patient at Glen Cove, having suffered a miscarriage.

Manny filled our apartment with flowers in an attempt to console me, but the only real consolation I had was my belief in a higher power. Everything had a reason for happening. There were no accidents. Our landlady, a surrogate mother, fixed my favorite filet mignon dinner. Ironically, her own daughter had been discharged from the same hospital that day after giving birth to a healthy baby girl while I walked out with empty arms. Later that night, I heard the newborn baby's cries through the apartment walls. Till then, I had never known the depth of my own sorrow.

But here was another important lesson: you may not get what you want, but God always gives you what you need.

CHAPTER FIFTEEN

Manhattan State Hospital

A few weeks before Manny and I began our new jobs, I received a letter from my father. It was a serious message, but tinged with irony. My father had suffered a pulmonary embolism, and according to him, the end was near. He wanted us to visit one last time. He also wanted me, his favorite doctor, the only one he trusted, to examine him. How hard we had fought over my desire to become a doctor!

After the miscarriage and the move, Manny and I were exhausted. We did not want to travel to Switzerland. But Seppli's last request had taught me never to ignore a dying patient. When they want to talk, they do not mean tomorrow. They want to talk immediately. So Manny sold his new Impala to pay for our airline tickets and three days later we walked into my father's hospital room. Instead of the deathbed scene we expected, we found my father out of bed, looking quite pink. The next day we took him home.

It was not like him to overreact. Neither was it like Manny not to say anything about having sold his car for nothing. Something was going on. Later on, I realized that my father, while hospitalized, must have had a premonition that we needed to repair our relationship before it was too late, which was exactly what happened. For the rest of the week, my father philosophized with me about life like never before. It made us closer than ever, and I think Manny realized that was worth far more than any car.

Once we returned to New York, I began my residency at

Manhattan State Hospital, where not as much value was placed on life. It was July 1959, one of those hot, sticky summer days. I had every right to feel uncomfortable as I entered the hospital. It was a frightening complex of brick buildings, home to hundreds of extremely disturbed, mentally ill people. They were the worst-case scenarios. Some spent twenty years and more there.

I could not believe what I saw. The place was packed beyond capacity with destitute people whose contorted faces, spasmodic gestures and anguished screams let you know they were living a real-life hell. Later that night, in my journal I described what I had seen as "a nightmare of bedlam." It might have been worse.

My unit was in a one-floor building, where forty chronic schizophrenic women lived. I was told they were hopeless. I observed only one thing to support that claim, the head nurse. She was a friend of the boss and thus made her own rules, which included allowing her precious cats to run freely around the unit. They left putrid odors in every corner. Because the windows were barred and shut, the place stank wretchedly. I instantly felt sorry for my co-workers, Dr. Philippe Trochu, a resident, and Grace Miller, a black social worker. Both were quality, caring individuals.

How they survived there was beyond me, though the patients had it many times worse. They were beaten with sticks, punished with electroshock treatments and on occasion placed in bathtubs which were then filled as high as their necks with hot water and then left there for up to twenty-four hours. Many were used as human guinea pigs in experiments with LSD, psilocybin and mescaline. If they protested—and all of them did—they were subjected to even more inhumane punishments.

As a researcher, I was thrown into the vortex of this snake pit. My official job was to record the effects of these experimental hallucinogenic drugs on patients, but after listening to a few of them recall the terrifying visions that resulted from the drugs, I vowed to end the practice and change the way the institute was run.

It would be easy to break the routines of the hospital or the patients. Most patients hovered in a corner of their room, or in the recreation room, without any occupation, distraction or stimulation. In the morning, they stood in line for medication that put them in a stupor and left them with horrible side effects. Later in the day, they followed a similar procedure. I realized there was a place for drugs like Thorazine in the treatment of psychotics, but most of these people were grossly overmedicated, victims of exaggerated detachment. Instead of drugs, they needed care and comfort.

With the help of my co-workers, I altered the routines designed to motivate patients to care for themselves. If they wanted Coca-Cola and cigarettes, they had to earn the money to pay for those privileges. They had to get out of bed on time, dress themselves, comb their hair and stand in line on time. Those who couldn't—or wouldn't—perform these simple tasks bore the consequences. They lost a day's income. After one week, everybody stood in line. On Friday night, I handed out their pay. Some drank all their Cokes and smoked all their cigarettes the first night. But we got results.

What did I know about psychiatry? Nothing. But I knew about life and I opened myself up to the misery, loneliness and fear these patients felt. If they talked to me, I talked back. If they shared their feelings, then I listened and replied. They sensed this, and suddenly they weren't so alone and fearful anymore.

I battled more with my boss than I did with the patients. He was against reducing their medications, even though I eventually introduced menial but productive work into their routines. Filling boxes with mascara pencils wasn't much, but it beat sitting around in drugged trances. Later on, I even took the well-behaved patients out on field trips. I taught them how to use the subway and purchase tokens, and on special occasions I even took them shopping at Macy's. My patients knew I cared and they got better.

At home, Manny heard all about my patients, including one young woman named Rachel. She was a catatonic schizophrenic, classified as one of the hopeless. For years, she had spent every day standing in exactly the same spot in the yard. No one could remember the last time she had spoken a word, or even made a sound. When I fought to get her transferred into my ward, people thought I was nuts.

But once she was under my care, I treated her like the others. I made her perform her tasks, and I made her stand in the group

117

when we celebrated Christmas, Chanukah and even her own birthday. After almost a year of attention, Rachel finally spoke. It happened during art therapy, as she drew a picture. A doctor looked at her work and she asked, "Do you like it?"

It was not long before Rachel left the hospital, got a place of her own and worked as a silk-screen artist.

I rejoiced with every success, large ones and small ones, such as when a man who always faced the wall decided to turn and look at the group. But then I faced a very difficult choice. In May, I was invited to reapply for the pediatrics program at Columbia Presbyterian. I debated whether to pursue my dream or stay with my patients. It was impossible to decide, but later that same week I found out I was pregnant again. That solved that problem.

At the end of June, though, I suffered another miscarriage. The fear of another miscarriage was why I had refused to let myself get excited about the pregnancy. I did not want to suffer the sadness and depression, even though that could not be helped. My obstetrician said that I was one of those women who lose their babies. I did not believe him, not when my dreams included a picture of me with children. I attributed the miscarriages to fate.

Instead I spent another year at Manhattan State Hospital, where my objective was to effect the discharge of as many of my patients as possible. I wanted to get the most functional patients jobs outside the hospital. They left in the morning, returned at night and learned how to use their money to buy basics other than Coke and cigarettes. My superiors noticed my success and asked for the theory behind my approach. I had none.

"I do whatever feels right after I get to know the patient," I explained. "You can't drug them into a torpor and hope they get better. You have to treat them like people.

"I don't refer to them the way you do," I continued. "I don't say, 'Oh, the schizophrenic in room so-and-so.' I know them by name. I know their habits. And they respond."

The greatest success resulted from the "open house" program Grace Miller and I started. Neighborhood families were invited to visit the hospital and adopt patients. In other words, we were generating relationships for people who were absolutely clueless about how to have any kind of relationship. Some patients

118

responded beautifully. They acquired a sense of responsibility and purpose to their lives. Some even learned to plan for future visits.

The most wondrous success of all was with a woman named Alice. Close to being discharged after twenty years in the mental ward, Alice shocked everybody one day with an unusual request. She wanted to see her children again. Children? None of us knew what she was talking about.

But Grace looked into the matter and discovered that Alice did indeed have two children. Both had been very young when she was committed. It turned out they had been told their mother had died.

My social worker colleague found those two children, now grown up, and told them about the hospital's "adoption" program. She said there was a "lonely old lady" who needed a surrogate family. In memory of their mother, they agreed. Neither was informed of the old lady's real identity. But I will never forget Alice's incredible smile when she faced the children she thought had forsaken her. Eventually, after Alice was released, the children made her part of their family . . . again.

Speaking of family, Manny and I kept on trying to start our own. In the fall of 1959, I got pregnant again. The baby was due in mid-June 1960. For nine months, Manny treated me like I was breakable. Somehow I knew the baby was going to take. Rather than worry about another miscarriage, I pictured a little boy or girl. I imagined how I would spoil it. When you thought about it, life was hard. Every day presented a new challenge. I wondered why anyone in her right mind wanted to bring another life into the world. But then I would think of all the beauty in the world and laugh. Why wouldn't you?

Manny and I moved to an apartment in the Bronx. It was larger than either of our other places. About a week before my due date, my mother flew over to help me with the baby, though she was not at all inconvenienced when I was late, since it gave her more time to spend in Macy's and the other department stores.

At three weeks past my delivery date, Manny and I began driving our car down cobblestone streets in Brooklyn. We actually *searched* for potholes to drive over. Ironically, we were stuck on the Long Island Expressway in a thunderstorm when I finally went into labor. Per our plan, we drove to Glen Cove Hospital. After fifteen hours of labor, I began making progress, though by that time the doctors had decided to take over using forceps. I was opposed to such procedures, but at that point I was too tired to care. I just wanted to hold a healthy baby.

All I remember is my own scream. Then a gorgeous, healthy child nestled in my arms, eyes open, searching the brand-new sights of the world. It was the most beautiful baby I had ever seen. I checked everything carefully. A little boy. My son. He weighed almost eight pounds, was topped by a mess of dark hair and had the most exquisite long, dark eyelashes any of us had ever seen on a child. Manny named him Kenneth. Neither I nor my mother could pronounce the "th" in his name very clearly, but we didn't care. We were thrilled by his arrival.

Manny and I had agreed to let our children decide questions of religion on their own when they were old enough, but he still insisted on a circumcision. "It's for my family," he said. But when I heard a rabbi was on his way, I imagined a circumcision and then a bar mitzvah, and that was too much for me.

Then Kenneth's pediatrician calmed my angst by reporting a medical problem. The baby was having trouble urinating; his foreskin was closed. He had to perform a circumcision immediately. Although groggy, I jumped out of bed faster than ever before and assisted the procedure.

I could not imagine being any happier. Tired, yes. Happier, never. I often marveled at how my own mother had managed with four children—three of whom arrived at once. But as mothers do, she said it was nothing out of the ordinary. She did not understand why I was going back to work. At the time, very few women managed to raise children and have a career. I guess I was one of those women who never saw the choice. My family was the most important thing in the world to me, but I also had to fulfill a calling.

After a month at home, I returned to Manhattan State Hospital, where I finished my second year of residency. My accomplishments included ending the most sadistic punishments and the discharge of 94 percent of my "hopeless" schizophrenics into productive, self-sufficient lives outside the hospital. Yet I still needed one more year of residency to become a full-fledged psychiatrist. The specialty still

120

didn't sound right to me, but both Manny and I agreed it was too late for me to start over.

I applied to Montefiore, a more sophisticated, intellectually stimulating institution than the state hospital, and was called in for an interview. It did not go well. My interrogator, a doctor with the personality of a cold fish, seemed intent only on humiliating me. His questions revealed my lack of knowledge about (and interest in) treating neurotics, alcoholics, sexually troubled individuals and other nonpsychotics; and the board allowed him to show off how much he knew. But he was only book smart.

To me, there was a big difference between what he knew from reading and what I had experienced at Manhattan State Hospital, and even though it meant risking my admission to Montefiore, I decided to tell him that. "Knowledge helps, but knowledge alone is not going to help anybody," I said. "If you do not use your head and your heart and your soul, you are not going to help a single human being."

That may not have answered any of his questions, but it made me feel a whole lot better.

CHAPTER SIXTEEN

Living Until Death

🐚

Shortly after I was accepted by Montefiore Hospital, where I was put in charge of the psychopharmacological clinic and also did liaison consulting for other departments, including neurology, I was asked by a neurologist to check on one of his patients. I spoke with the patient, a man in his twenties, who was supposedly suffering from psychosomatic paralysis and depression, and determined instead that he was in the later stages of ALS, or amyotrophic lateral sclerosis, an incurable degenerative disorder.

"The patient is preparing himself to die," I reported.

The neurologist not only disagreed; he ridiculed my diagnosis and argued that the patient just needed some tranquilizers to cure his morbid state of mind.

Yet days later the patient died.

My honesty was contrary to the way medicine was typically practiced in hospitals. But after a few months on the job I noticed that many doctors routinely avoided the mention of anything to do with death. Dying patients were treated as badly as my psychiatric patients at the state hospital. They were shunned and abused. Nobody was honest with them. A cancer patient might ask, "Am I dying?" and the doctor would reply, "Oh, don't be silly." That was not me.

But then I do not think Montefiore, or many other hospitals, had seen many doctors like me. Few had experience like my relief work in the war-torn villages of Europe, and even fewer were mothers, as I was to my baby son Kenneth. Plus my work with schizophrenic patients had showed me there was a curative power beyond drugs, beyond science, and that is what I brought each day to the hospital wards.

During my consultations, I sat on beds, held hands and talked for hours. There was, I learned, not a single dying human being who did not yearn for love, touch or communication. Dying patients did not want a safe distance from their doctors. They craved honesty. Even the most suicidally depressed patients could often, though not always, be convinced there was still meaning left in their lives. "Tell me what you're going through," I would say. "It will help me to help other people."

But, tragically, the worst cases—those people in the last stages of illness, those who were in the process of dying—were given the worst treatment. They were put in the rooms farthest from the nursing stations. They were forced to lie under bright lights they could not shut off. They were denied visitors, except during prescribéd hours. They were left alone to die, as if death might be contagious.

I refused to go along with such practices. They seemed wrong to me. So I stayed with my dying patients for however long it took, and I told them I would.

Although I worked all over the hospital, I gravitated toward those cases considered the worst—dying patients. They were the best teachers I ever had. I observed them struggling to accept fate. I listened to them lash out at God. I shrugged helplessly when they cried out, "Why me?" I heard them make peace with Him. I noticed that if there was another human being who cared, they would arrive at a point of acceptance. These were what I would eventually describe as the different stages of dying, though they apply to the way we deal with any type of loss.

By listening, I came to know that all dying patients know they are dying. It's not a question of "Do we tell him?" or "Does he know?"

The only question to ask is: "Can I hear him?'

Halfway around the world my own father was trying to get someone to listen to him. In September, my mother called to inform us that my father was in the hospital, dying. She assured me that it was not a false alarm this time. Manny could get no

124

time off, but I took Kenneth and left on the first plane the next day.

At the hospital, I saw that he was dying. He had septicemia, a deadly infection that was due to a botched operation on his elbow. My father was attached to machines suctioning pus from his abdomen. He was thin and in pain. Medicine was not helping anymore. All my father wanted was to go home. Nobody heard him. His doctor refused to discharge him, and so did the hospital.

But my father threatened to commit suicide if he was not allowed to die in the peace and comfort of his own home. My mother was so weary and distraught that she was threatening to join him. I knew the story that no one was talking about. My father's father, who had broken his spine, died in a nursing home. His last wish had been to be taken home. But my father had refused, listening to doctors instead. Now he was in practically the same situation.

No one in the hospital cared that I was a doctor. They said I could take him home if I signed a paper releasing them from responsibility.

"The trip will probably kill him," his doctor warned.

I looked at my father in bed, helpless, suffering pain and wanting to go home. The choice was mine. At that moment, I remembered how he had rescued me when I had slipped into a crevice while hiking across a glacier. If not for the rope he taught me how to tie, I would have fallen to my death in the abyss. Now I was going to rescue him.

I signed the paper.

My stubborn father, having gotten his own way, wanted to celebrate. He asked for a glass of his favorite wine, which I'd sneaked into his room a few days earlier. While helping him hold the glass to his lips, I noticed the wine, drop by drop, come out of one of the many tubes in his body. I knew then it was time to let him go.

After sickroom equipment was set up, we brought my father home. I sat next to him in the ambulance, noticing how his mood brightened as we neared the house. Periodically he squeezed my hand to let me know how much he appreciated this effort. As the ambulance attendants carried him to his bedroom, I saw how shriveled his once-powerful body had become. But he bossed everyone around until he was at last set down in his own bed. Finally he whispered, "Home at last."

For the next two days he dozed peacefully. During conscious moments, he gazed at pictures of his beloved mountains or his skiing trophies. My mother and I kept a constant vigil by his bedside. For some reason I do not remember, my siblings were unable to make it home, but they kept in touch. A nurse had been hired, though I took the responsibility for making sure he was clean and comfortable. It reminded me that nursing was really strenuous work.

As he neared the end, my father refused to eat. It was too painful. But he asked for different bottles of wine from his cellar. It was in character.

On the last night, I watched him sleep in excruciating pain. At some critical point, I even gave him an injection of morphine. But then the next afternoon the most extraordinary thing happened. My father awoke from his troubled sleep and asked me to open the window so he could hear the church bells more clearly. For a few moments we listened to the familiar chimes of the Kreuzkirche. Then my father began conversing with his own father, apologizing for letting him die in that dreadful nursing home.

"Perhaps I've paid with all my present suffering," he said, and then he promised to see him soon.

In the midst of their talk, my father had turned and asked me for a glass of water. I marveled that he was clearly oriented and able to shift back and forth from one reality to another. Naturally I could not see or hear my grandfather. Apparently my father took care of a lot of unfinished business. Later that night, he weakened significantly. I slept on a cot right beside him. In the morning, I made sure he was comfortable, kissed his warm forehead, clasped his hand and then sneaked into the kitchen for a cup of coffee. I was gone two minutes. When I came back my father was dead.

For the next half hour my mother and I sat beside him, saying our goodbyes. He had been a great man, but he was no longer there. Whatever it was that had made my father him—energy, spirit and mind—was gone. His soul had taken flight from his physical body. I was certain his own father had guided him straight into heaven, where surely he was embraced by the unconditional love of God. I had no knowledge yet of life after death, but I was sure my father was finally at peace.

What next? I notified the proper city health office, which would not only remove the corpse but also supply free of charge the casket and limousine for the funeral. The nurse I'd hired inexplicably took off once she heard my father had died, leaving the final care of his body to me. A friend of mine, Dr. Bridgette Willisau, generously helped. Together we washed the pus and stool off my father's deteriorated body, then carefully dressed him in a nice suit. We worked in a kind of religious silence, and I reflected gratefully that my father had gotten a chance to see Kenneth, and that my son had known his grandfather, if only for a short time. I'd never known any of my grandparents.

By the time the two health officials arrived with a casket, my father was dressed and lying on the bed in a clean and tidy room. After they gently placed him in the casket, one of the men took me aside and discreetly, in a whisper, asked if I wanted to get some flowers from the garden and put them in my father's hands. How did he know? How could I have forgotten? It was my father who stimulated my love of flowers, who opened my eyes to the beauty of nature. I ran downstairs holding Kenneth, picked the loveliest chrysanthemums we could find and put them in my father's hands.

The funeral was three days later. In the same chapel where his daughters were married, my father was remembered by people he worked with, students he taught and friends from the Ski Club. Except for my brother, the entire family attended the service, which concluded with his favorite hymns. Our grieving lasted awhile longer, but none of us were left with any regrets. Later that night in my journal I wrote, "My father truly lived until he died."

CHAPTER SEVENTEEN

My First Lecture

By 1962, I had become Americanized. Four years did that to me. I chewed gum, I ate hamburgers and sugary breakfast cereals and I supported Kennedy over Nixon. I prepared my mother for one of her visits with a letter that warned, "Don't be too shocked to hear that I wear pants as often as skirts when I go out."

But I was still bothered by a restlessness that I could not explain, an inner sense that, despite marriage and motherhood, I was not settled in life. Not yet. I tried understanding it in my journal, where I wrote, "I still don't know why I'm in America, but there has to be a reason. I know there is a frontier out there, and that sometime I shall be traveling into the unknown territory."

I have no idea what made me feel that way, but that summer, just as I predicted, I traveled to the West. Manny and I found positions at the University of Colorado, the only medical school in the country that had openings in both neuropathology and psychiatry. We drove to Denver in Manny's brand-new convertible. My mother traveled with us, helping care for Kenneth. The scenery was so grand and beautiful and wide open. It really stirred up my passion for Mother Nature.

Once in Denver, we found that our house was not quite ready. It was no problem. We parked the U-Haul trailer in the driveway and took off on a sightseeing trip. We visited Manny's brother in Los Angeles, and then, only because my mother, who was new to map reading, swore that Mexico was "right next door," we drove to Tijuana. On the return, I suggested heading toward the juncture where Arizona, Utah, Colorado and New Mexico all intersected, the Four Corners area.

It was a great choice that allowed us to gaze at the large mesas, buttes and rocks at Monument Valley. I felt an eerie familiarity there, especially when I spotted an Indian woman riding on horseback off in the distance. The scene was so familiar, as though I had seen it before, and then with a shiver of excitement I recalled my dream on the ship the night before we arrived in America. I did not tell Manny or my mother, but that night I sat in bed and let my mind ask questions, no matter how far-out they seemed. Then, so I would not forget, I got out my journal and wrote.

> I know very little about the philosophy of reincarnation. I've always tended to associate reincarnation with way-out people debating their former lives in incense-filled rooms. That's not been my kind of upbringing. I'm at home in laboratories. But I know now there are mysteries of the mind, the psyche, the spirit that cannot be probed by microscopes or chemical reactions. In time I'll know more. In time I'll understand.

In Denver, it was back to reality, where I searched for a purpose to my life. That was particularly true at the hospital. I was a psychiatrist, but regular psychiatry was definitely not for me. I also tried working with troubled adults and children. But what ended up capturing my interest was the type of intuitive psychiatry I had practiced on schizophrenics at Manhattan State Hospital, a nontraditional one-on-one type of interaction, rather than medication and group sessions. I talked about it with my university colleagues, but none of them offered any encouragement.

What was I going to do with myself? I asked three distinguished psychiatrists, men with great reputations, for advice. They suggested undergoing analysis at the famous Psychoanalytic Institute in Chicago, a traditional answer that was not really practical for my life at the time.

Then I sat in on a lecture given by Professor Sydney Margolin, the respected chief of the psychiatric department's new psychophysiology laboratory. Professor Margolin commanded attention from the podium. He was an older man with long gray hair who spoke with a thick Austrian accent. He was a riveting speaker, a great performer. After listening for only a few minutes, I knew he was exactly my cup of tea.

Not surprisingly Professor Margolin's lectures were very popular. I attended several. He kind of materialized onstage. The topics of his lectures were always a surprise. Eventually I followed him into his office and introduced myself. He was friendly and I soon found him more fascinating in person. We spoke for a long time, in German and English. Like one of his lectures, we were all over the map. In between, I discussed my personal quandary and he talked about his interest in the Ute Indian tribe.

Unlike his colleagues, he did not mention going to Chicago. Instead he encouraged me to take a position in his lab. I accepted.

Professor Margolin was a difficult, demanding boss, but his work on psychosomatic illness was the most fulfilling work I had done in Denver. Sometimes all I did was organize the odd electronic equipment the professor had salvaged from other departments. But that was okay. He was unconventional. For instance, his lab team included an electrician, a good handyman and a devoted secretary. The lab itself teemed with machines—polygraphs, EKGs and so on. Professor Margolin was interested in measuring the relationship between a patient's thoughts and emotions and pathology. He also used hypnosis and he believed in reincarnation.

My happiness at work carried over to my home life. Manny was also pleased with his role as an important lecturer in the neuropathology department. Our home was everything that I imagined family life should be. Outside I made a Swiss rock garden, including a spruce tree, alpine flowers and my first U.S. edelweiss. On weekends, we took Kenneth to the zoo and hiked through the Rockies. Socially we spent many delightful evenings with Professor Margolin and his wife, listening to classical music and debating topics from Freud to past-life theories.

The disappointments were few, but significant to our family. In 1964, our second year in Denver, I was pregnant twice. Each time, I suffered a miscarriage. It was increasingly difficult to deal with the frustration, rather than the loss. Both Manny and I wanted to add another child to our brood. I wanted two children. I had my boy. If God was kind, I would also have a girl. I was going to keep trying.

Professor Margolin traveled frequently, and one day he called me into his office to tell me he was leaving for Europe in two weeks. I thought he simply wanted to discuss various cities and sites, as we often did when reminiscing about our well-traveled youths. Not today, though. In his typical unpredictable manner, the professor appointed me to take over his lectures at the medical school. It took a moment for his request to sink in, but then almost instantly I broke out in a nervous sweat.

This wasn't just an honor; it was an impossibility. Professor Margolin was a colorful, animated speaker whose lectures were more like performances, intellectual one-man productions. They attracted the largest audiences in the school. How could I step into those shoes? When it came to speaking in front of groups, large or small, I was terribly shy and insecure. "You have two weeks to prepare," he said reassuringly. "I don't follow a syllabus. If you'd like, look through my files. Pick any topic you want."

Necessity followed panic. For the next week, I planted myself in the library and plowed through book after book, trying to find an original topic. I wasn't a fan of conventional psychiatry. Nor did I approve of all the drugs patients were given to make them "manageable." And I also crossed out anything too specialized, such as anything about different psychoses. After all, most of the students who'd be listening were interested in specialties other than psychiatry.

But I had to fill two hours, and I wanted a topic that satisfied my expectations of what future physicians needed to know about psychiatry. What would interest an orthopedic surgeon? A urologist? My experiences had taught me that most doctors were far too detached in their approach to patients. They desperately needed to confront the simple, down-to-earth feelings, fears and defenses that people had when they entered the hospital. They needed to treat patients as fellow human beings.

So what, I asked myself, was the ground everyone had in

common? No matter how much literature I looked at, nothing came to mind.

Then one day the subject popped into my mind. Death. Every patient and doctor thought about it. Most feared it. Sooner or later, everybody had to confront it. It was something doctors and patients had in common, and it was probably the greatest mystery in medicine. The biggest taboo too.

That became my topic. I tried doing research. But the library did not have any material, except for a difficult, academic psychoanalytic treatise and a few sociological studies on the death rituals of Buddhists, Jews, American Indians and others. I intended a far different approach. My thesis was the simple idea that doctors would be more comfortable dealing with death if they understood it better, if they simply talked about what it was like to die.

Well, I was on my own. Professor Margolin always divided his lectures into two parts: the first hour was a theoretical talk; the second hour presented empirical evidence supporting what he had said earlier. I worked harder than ever preparing for the first hour, but then I realized that I had to invent something for the second hour.

What?

I walked through the hospital for a few days, searching and thinking and hoping something would pop into my head. While on my rounds one day, I sat with a sixteen-year-old girl who was dying of leukemia, talking, as we had several times previously, about her situation. All of a sudden it dawned on me that Linda was very direct, comfortable and focused discussing her condition. Her doctor's impersonal treatment drained whatever hope she had, but she also freely and eloquently expressed her anger toward her family, who weren't coping well with her dying. Her mother had recently advertised her daughter's plight, asking the public to send in "Happy Sweet Sixteen" birthday cards for what was sure to be the girl's last birthday.

On the day we talked, an enormous bag of birthday greetings had been delivered. They were well-meaning but impersonal, written by total strangers. But in our conversation, Linda shoved the mail aside with her thin, frail arms. Then her pallid cheeks flushed with anger as she admitted wanting instead meaningful,

133

caring visits from her family and relatives. "I wish they'd think about how I feel!" she fumed. "I mean, why me? Why did God pick me to die?"

She fascinated me, this brave girl, and I knew the medical students had to hear from her. "Tell them all the things you could never tell your mother," I urged. "Tell them what it's like to be sixteen and to be dying. If you are furious, get it out. Use any kind of language you want. Just talk from the heart and soul."

On the day of the lecture, I stood at the podium in the large amphitheater and read from my neatly typed notes. Maybe it was my accent, but the response was nothing like the one Professor Margolin received. The students behaved inexcusably badly. They chewed gum, talked among themselves and were basically disrespectful and rude. Although I plowed ahead with my speech, I wondered if any of the students could've lectured in French or German. I also thought about the Swiss medical schools where professors commanded the highest respect from students. No one would dare chew gum or whisper in class. But I was thousands of miles from my former home.

I was also so involved in getting through my lecture that I didn't notice the class got quieter and more behaved as I neared the end of the first hour. By then I was calm and looking forward to surprising my students in the second half with an actual dying patient. During the break, I fetched my daring sixteen-year-old, who had dressed nicely and done her hair, and wheeled her to the center of the auditorium's stage. Whereas I had been a nervous wreck an hour earlier, Linda's clear brown eyes and determined jaw indicated that she was perfectly calm, composed and ready.

As the students returned from the break, they quietly and nervously took their seats, while I introduced the girl and explained that she had generously volunteered to answer their questions on what it was like to be terminally ill. There was the slight, nervous rustle of people shifting in their chairs and then a quiet so deep it was disturbing. Obviously the students were uncomfortable. When I asked for volunteers, nobody raised a hand. Finally I selected a handful of students, called them onto the stage and instructed them to ask questions. All they could muster were questions about her blood count, the size of her liver, her reaction to chemotherapy and other clinical details.

When it was clear they weren't going to ask anything about her personal feelings, I decided to steer the interview in the direction I envisioned. But I didn't have to. In a passionate fit of anger, Linda herself lost patience with her interrogators. Fixing her unimpressed brown eyes on them, she posed and answered the questions she had always wanted her physician and team of specialists to ask her. What was it like to be sixteen and given only a few weeks to live? What was it like not to be able to dream about the high school prom? Or go on a date? Or not worry about growing up and choosing a profession? Or a husband? What helps you make it through each day? Why won't people tell you the truth?

After nearly half an hour, Linda tired and returned to her bed, leaving the students in a stunned, emotional, almost reverential silence. Quite a change had overtaken them. Although the lecture time was over, no one got up to leave. They wanted to talk but didn't know what to say until I started the discussion. Most admitted that Linda had moved them to tears. Finally I suggested that their reactions, while instigated by the dying girl, were in fact due to an admission of their own fragile mortality. For the first time, most of them confronted feelings and fears about the possibility, and inevitability, of their own death. They couldn't help but think about what it would be like if they were in Linda's place.

"Now you are reacting like human beings instead of scientists," I offered.

Silence.

"Maybe now you'll not only know how a dying patient feels, but you'll also be able to treat them with compassion, the same compassion that you'd want for yourself."

Drained by the lecture, I sipped coffee in my office and found myself thinking back to a laboratory accident that happened in Zurich in 1943. While I was mixing some chemicals in the lab, a bottle dropped and burst into flames. My face, hands and head were badly burned. I spent two excruciatingly painful weeks in the hospital, unable to talk or move my hands, while each day doctors tortured me as they ripped off old bandages as well as my tender skin, burned out my wounds with silver nitrate and then rebandaged me. They predicted I'd never regain full mobility of my fingers.

But a lab technician friend who tiptoed into my room at night without my doctor's knowledge rigged up a contraption that used increasing increments of weight to slowly exercise my fingers. It was our secret. A week before being discharged, the doctor brought in a group of medical students to look at me. As he explained the case and why my fingers were useless, I stifled a strong desire to grin and then suddenly raised my hand and flexed and bent my fingers, leaving them speechless. "How?" he asked.

I shared my secret, and I think everybody learned something in the process. Their thinking was forever changed.

Just a few hours earlier, sixteen-year-old Linda had done the same for a bunch of medical students. She had taught them, as I was also learning, what was relevant and valuable at the end of life and what wasted too much of our time and energy. Indeed, the lessons of her short life resonated for many years after she died.

There was an enormous amount to learn about life by listening to dying patients.

*

CHAPTER EIGHTEEN

Motherhood

{&

For the half dozen lectures I gave, which included topics other than death, I worked with a sense of purpose. When Professor Margolin returned I felt it wane. I craved it badly enough to finally apply to Chicago's Psychoanalytic Institute, even though the thought of spending hours each day in psychoanalysis was enough to make me hate myself. I knew how wrong it was when my application was accepted in early 1963. But then I had the perfect excuse to turn it down—I found out I was pregnant.

As with Kenneth, I sensed that this baby would make it through the full term. Still, I took no chances. I even underwent a minor surgical procedure, which my obstetrician said was necessary to "keep the baby in the oven." But for nine months, I was in peak health, physically and emotionally. I had no trouble balancing work, where I ran an inpatient unit for highly disturbed people, and home. Kenneth, an energetic and happy three-year-old shared the excitement of a new brother or sister.

On December 5, 1963, my water broke. I had just finished giving a lecture. It was too early to go into labor, but I sat down at my desk and asked a student to call Manny. Since he worked in the same building, he arrived within minutes. Although I felt perfectly fine, no different than before, he took me home and called the obstetrician. My OB was not particularly concerned and told me to rest and come into his office on Monday. "Just stay in bed, control your temperature and don't exert yourself," he said.

Easy for a man to say. If I were to be admitted to the hospital on Monday, I needed to make some preparations. I spent the weekend freezing meals for Manny and Kenneth and packing clothes in a suitcase. On Monday morning, I still felt okay but my abdominal wall was rock hard when I waddled into the obstetrician's office. My doctor was alarmed and frightened by this irregular condition. He diagnosed it as peritonitis, a life-threatening infection that could have been avoided if I'd been seen the day my water broke.

I was rushed to the nearby Catholic hospital, where nuns prepared to induce labor, while my doctor informed me that the baby would likely be too small to survive. "It certainly won't tolerate any pain medication," he said. As he said this, I was already suffering extreme pain. One simple touch to my stomach caused excruciating pain, wave after wave, till I was consumed by it.

I noticed that the nuns had prepared a table with holy water and the paraphernalia needed for baptism. I knew what that meant. They expected the baby to die. Instead of being concerned about me and my health, they wanted to make sure they could baptize the newborn before it died.

For forty-eight hours, I rode waves of pain in and out of con-sciousness. Manny sat next to me, but there was nothing he could to do to help me make progress. I nearly stopped breathing once, and several other times I thought I was dying. Toward the end, the doctor finally attempted a spinal injection to help me with the pain. But nothing worked. Whatever was going to happen had to happen naturally. Finally, after two days of pain, I heard the cry of a newborn baby. Then someone said, "It's a girl!"

Although everyone had expected a stillborn baby, Barbara was very much alive and fighting to remain so. She weighed slightly more than three pounds. I studied her face briefly before a nun whisked her off to an incubator. Later I would point out the similarity to my own birth as a "two-pound nothing" who wasn't expected to survive. But then, exhausted by the constant pain, I had barely enough energy to smile at the birth of the little girl I desperately wanted, before falling into a deep and satisfied sleep.

After three days in the hospital, I went home. Sadly I was not allowed to bring my daughter with me. Since she was having trouble gaining weight, the doctors thought she should remain in the hospital till she got stronger. For the next week, I drove there every three hours to nurse her. The pediatricians did not like it when I said that I could take better care of my baby at home, but finally, after seven days, I put on my white lab coat and checked Barbara out of the hospital myself.

Now the picture was complete. I had a home, a husband and my beautiful Kenneth and Barbara. The work at home multiplied. But I remember being in the kitchen one evening and seeing Kenneth rocking his little sister on his knee. Manny was in his chair, reading. My little world seemed in order.

But then Manny, the only neuropathologist in Denver, grew restless. His ambition was not being satisfied there and he craved more intellectual stimulation. I understood and told him to look around for another position. I would go wherever he found the best opportunity for both of us. In the spring of 1965, I took the children on a vacation to Switzerland, and when we got back Manny had found positions for each of us in either Albuquerque, New Mexico, or Chicago. The choice was not difficult to make.

At the start of summer, we moved to Chicago. Actually, we found a modern, two-story home in Marynook, a middle-class, racially integrated suburb. Manny accepted a good offer from Northwestern University Medical Center while I joined the psychiatric department at Billings Hospital, which was associated with the University of Chicago, and arranged to begin analysis at the Psychoanalytic Institute.

Analysis was not something I looked forward to. I conveniently forgot about it until the phone rang one day while I was emptying moving boxes. I heard a rather authoritarian, arrogant male voice. It was a turnoff already. The caller then informed me that my first session with an analyst handpicked by the institute was scheduled for the next Monday.

I explained that we had just moved and didn't have a baby-sitter yet, so the timing was not great. But he wasn't interested in excuses.

It went downhill from there. At my first session, I was kept waiting forty-five minutes. Once my analyst asked me into his office, I sat down and waited for his instructions. Nothing happened. The time passed in stiff, agonizing silence. The analyst just glared at me unhappily. I felt as if I was being tortured.

Finally, he asked, "Do you plan to just sit there in silence?"

Taking that as my cue, I made an effort to talk about my early life and the difficulties of having been born a triplet. But after several minutes, he stopped me. He said he couldn't understand a single word I had uttered and concluded that my problem was an obvious one. I had a speech impediment. "I don't know why the institute considered you for a training analysis," he said. "You can't even speak."

Enough of that. I walked out and slammed the door behind me. Later that night he called me at home and begged me to come back for another session, if only to give closure to our mutual dislike. For some crazy reason, I agreed. But the second session lasted even less time than the first. I decided that we simply didn't like each other and there was no sense wasting time trying to figure out why.

I did not give up on analysis, though. After asking for recommendations, I finally settled into a routine with Dr. Helmut Baum. It lasted thirty-nine months. I eventually realized there was some value to analysis. I got some new insight into my personality, why I was so headstrong and independent.

Still, I did not become a fan of classic psychiatry, including the heavily publicized pharmaceutical breakthroughs of my department. I felt drugs were relied on much too frequently. I thought that a patient's social, cultural and family background was not given enough consideration. I also complained about the emphasis on publishing scientific papers and the stature that accorded. It did not seem to me that dealing with patients and their problems was considered as important as the academics behind it.

That is no doubt why my first love was working with medical students. They were all eager and open to learning. They were interested in discussing new ideas, opinions, attitudes and research projects. They ate up case studies. They wanted experiences of their own. They needed mothering. In a short time, my office became a magnet for such students, who spread the word that there was a place on campus where you could air your thoughts and problems to a patient and understanding ear. It seemed as if I heard every conceivable question. But then I got one that showed me why it was no accident that I was in Chicago.

CHAPTER NINETEEN

On Death and Dying

My life was a juggling act that would have frightened Freud and Jung. In addition to braving downtown Chicago traffic, finding a housekeeper, battling Manny for permission to have my own checking account and shopping for groceries, I prepared my lectures and served as the psychiatric liaison to other departments. At times I felt as if there was no way I could handle any more responsibilities.

But one day in the fall of 1965 there was a knock on my office door. Four men from Chicago's Theological Seminary introduced themselves and said they were researching a paper whose thesis proposed that death was the ultimate crisis people had to deal with. They had somehow gotten a transcript of my first lecture in Denver, but someone had told them that I had also written a paper, which they had been unable to find, and thus they came directly to me.

They were disappointed when I told them that no such paper existed, but I invited them to sit down and talk. I was not surprised seminary students were interested in the subject of death and dying. They had as much reason to study death and dying as any doctor. They dealt with dying patients too. Certainly they had their own questions about death and dying that could not be answered by reading the Bible.

During our talk, the seminary students admitted a helplessness and confusion when it came to what they would say to people who asked questions about death and dying. None of .

them had ever talked with a dying person or seen a dead body. They wondered if I had any ideas on how they could get such practical experience. They even suggested observing when I visited with a dying patient. Little did I know they were supplying the impetus for my work on death and dying.

Over the next week, I thought about how my psychiatric liaison work brought me into contact with patients from oncology, internal medicine and gynecology. Some patients suffered from terminal illnesses; others sat alone battling anxiety while waiting for radiation treatments or chemotherapy or just a simple X ray. But all of them were frightened, confused, lonely and desperately wanted another person there to share in their concerns. I did that naturally. I asked one question and it was like opening a floodgate.

So I surveyed the wards on my rounds for a dying patient who would be willing to speak to the theology students. I asked several other physicians if they had any dying patients, but they reacted with disgust. The doctor who supervised the ward with most of the terminal patients not only refused me permission to speak to any of his patients, he reprimanded me for trying to "exploit them." Few doctors then even admitted that their patients were dying, so what I was suggesting was pretty radical. I should probably have been more delicate and politic.

Finally one physician pointed to an elderly man on his ward. The man was dying of emphysema. The doctors said something like, "Try that one. You can't harm him." I immediately walked into the man's room and approached his bed. He was attached to breathing tubes and was obviously weak. But he was perfect. I asked if he would mind if I brought four students in the next day to ask him questions about how he was feeling at this point in his life. I felt that he understood my mission. But he suggested bringing them right away. "No," I said. "I'll bring them tomorrow."

My first mistake was not listening to what he told me. He had tried to let me know that time was short. I did not hear.

The next day I brought the four seminary students into his room, but he had gotten even weaker, too weak to say more than a word or two. He recognized me, though, and acknowledged our presence by pressing his hand to mine. A tear rolled down his cheek. "Thank you for trying," he whispered. After sitting with him a few moments, I took the students back to my office. We arrived there just about the same time that I got a message telling me that the old man had died.

I felt so lousy that I had put my own agenda ahead of the patient's. That old man had died without ever being able to share with another human what he was so eager to discuss the day before. Eventually I found another patient who was willing to speak to my seminary students. But that first lesson was a hard one, one I never forgot.

Perhaps the biggest obstacle anyone faces in the effort to understand death is that it's impossible for the unconscious mind to imagine an end to its own life. The only aspect it could understand was a sudden, frightening interruption of life, a tragic killing, a murder, one of several gruesome diseases. In other words, horrible pain. In a physician's mind, death meant something else. It meant failure. I could not help but observe how everybody at the hospital avoided the subject of death.

In this modern hospital, dying was a sad, lonely and impersonal event. Terminally ill patients were routed to back rooms. In the emergency room, patients lay in total isolation while doctors and their families debated whether or not they should be told what was wrong. To me, only one question ever needed asking: "How do we share the information?" If someone had asked me what the ideal situation was for a dying patient, I would have gone back to my childhood and described the death of the farmer who had gone home to be with family and friends. Truth was always the best.

The great advances in medicine had convinced people that life should be pain-free. Since death was only associated with pain, people avoided it. Adults rarely mentioned anything about it. Children were sent into other rooms when it was unavoidable. But facts are facts. Death was a part of life, the most important part of life. Physicians who were brilliant at prolonging life did not understand death was a part of it. If you did not have a good life, including the final moments, then you could not have a good death.

The need to explore these issues on an academic, scientific level was as great as it was inevitable that the responsibility would land

143

on my shoulders. Like those of my mentor Professor Margolin, my lectures on schizophrenia and other mental illnesses were considered both unorthodox and popular at the medical school. My experience with the four theology students was discussed by the more daring and inquisitive students. Shortly before Christmas, a half dozen students from the medical and theology schools asked if I would arrange another interview with a dying patient.

I agreed to try, and by the first half of 1967, six months later, I was leading one seminar every Friday. Not a single member of the hospital's faculty attended, which reflected their feelings toward the seminars, but they were hugely popular with medical and theology students as well as a surprising number of nurses, priests, rabbis and social workers. To accommodate the standing-room-only numbers, I moved the seminar into a large teaching auditorium, although my actual interview with the dying patient was conducted in a smaller room outfitted with a two-way mirror and an audio system so there was at least the illusion of privacy.

Every Monday I began searching for a single patient. It was never easy, since most doctors regarded me as sick and the seminars as exploitative. My more diplomatic colleagues gave excuses why their patients weren't good candidates. Most simply forbade me to talk with their critically ill patients. One afternoon I had a group of priests and nurses in my office when the phone rang and a doctor's loud, angry voice raged through the receiver: "How do you have the nerve to talk to Mrs. K. about dying when she does not even know how sick she is and may go home once more?"

Quite the point. Doctors who avoided my work and seminars usually had patients who unfortunately had difficulties coping with their illnesses. Since the physicians were so blocked about their own issues, the patients had no chance of ever discussing their concerns.

My goal was to break through the layer of professional denial that prohibited the patients from airing their innermost concerns. I remember one frustrating search for a suitable patient to interview, which I've written about before. Doctor after doctor informed me that no one on their wards was dying. Then I spotted an elderly gentleman in the hallway who was reading a paper headlined: "Old Soldiers Never Die." From appearances, I determined that his health was declining and asked if he was bothered reading about such subjects. He gave me a disdainful look as if I was like the other doctors who preferred not to deal with reality. Well, he ended up being a great subject.

Looking back, I think gender added to the resistance I encountered. As a woman who'd suffered four miscarriages and given birth to two healthy children, I accepted death as part of life's natural cycle. I had no other choice. It was unavoidable. It was the risk one assumed when giving birth as well as the risk one accepted simply for being alive. Yet the majority of doctors were men, and all but a few viewed death as a kind of failure.

In these earliest days of what would become known as the birth of thanatology—or the study of death—my greatest teacher was a black cleaning woman. I do not remember her name, but I saw her regularly in the halls, both day and night, depending on our shifts. But what drew my attention was the effect she had on many of the most seriously ill patients. Each time she left their rooms, there was, I noticed, a tangible difference in their attitudes.

I wanted to know her secret. Desperately curious, I literally spied on this woman who had never finished high school but knew a big secret.

Then one day our paths crossed in the hallway. Suddenly I was coaching myself to do what I always told my students to do: "For heaven's sake, when you have a question, ask it." Summoning all my courage, I walked directly up to this cleaning woman, a confrontational sort of approach, which I'm sure startled her, and without any subtlety or charm I literally blurted out, "What are you doing with my dying patients?"

Naturally, she became defensive. "I'm only cleaning the floors," she said politely, and then walked away.

"That's not what I'm talking about," I said too late.

For the next couple of weeks, we snooped around each other suspiciously. It was almost like a game. Finally, one afternoon she confronted me in the hallway and then pulled me behind the nursing station. It was a sight—this white-clad assistant professor of psychiatry being dragged off by this humble black cleaning woman. When we were completely alone, where no one could hear us, she bared her life's tragic history as well as her heart and soul in a way that was beyond my comprehension.

From Chicago's South Side, she grew up amid poverty and misery. Her home was a tenement where there was neither heat nor hot water and children were always malnourished and sick. Like most impoverished people, she had no defenses against illness or hunger. Children filled their aching bellies with cheap oatmeal, and doctors were for other people. One day her three-year-old son got very sick with pneumonia. She took him to the emergency room at the local hospital, but was turned away because she owed ten dollars. Desperate, she walked to Cook County Hospital, where they had to take indigent people.

There, unfortunately, she ran into a roomful of people like herself, people seriously in need of medical care. She was instructed to wait. But after three hours of sitting and waiting her turn, she watched her little boy wheeze and gasp and then die while she cradled him in her arms.

Although it was impossible not to feel the loss, I was struck more by the manner in which this woman told her story. While deeply sad, she had no negativity, no blame or bitterness or resentment. Instead there was a peacefulness to her demeanor that startled me. It was so odd, and I was so naive then, that I nearly asked, "Why are you telling me all this? What does it have to do with my dying patients?" But she looked at me with her dark, kind, understanding eyes and answered as if she was a mind reader. "You see, death is not a stranger to me. He is an old, old acquaintance."

Now I was the student looking at the teacher. "I'm not afraid of him anymore," she continued in her quiet, calm and direct tone. "Sometimes I walk into the rooms of these patients and they are simply petrified and have no one to talk to. So I go near them. Sometimes I even touch their hands and tell them not to worry, that it's not so terrible." She was then silent.

Not long after, I promoted this woman from cleaning woman to my first assistant. She provided the support I needed when it did not come from anyone else. That alone became a lesson that I have tried to pass along. You do not need special gurus or Babas to grow. Teachers come in all forms and disguises. Children, the terminally ill, a cleaning woman. All the theories and science in

146

the world could not help anyone as much as one human unafraid to open his heart to another.

Thank goodness for those few understanding doctors who permitted me access to their dying patients. Those introductory visits all followed the same simple routine. Wearing my white lab coat, which displayed my name and title, "Psychiatric Liaison," I asked permission to question them in front of my students about their illness, hospitalization and any other issues on their mind. I never used the words "death" and "dying" till they brought them up. Nothing but their name, age and diagnosis mattered to me. Usually the patient agreed to participate within a few minutes. In fact, I can't remember anyone ever refusing.

The auditorium usually filled to capacity thirty minutes before the lecture's scheduled start. A few minutes beforehand, I personally brought the patient on a stretcher or wheelchair into the interviewing room. Before we began, I stepped to the side for a moment to quietly ask that no harm come to the patient and that my questions enable him to share what he needed to share. It was like the Alcoholics Anonymous Prayer:

> *God grant me the serenity*
> *to accept the things I cannot change,*
> *the courage to change the things I can,*
> *and the wisdom to know the difference.*

Once the patients started to speak—and for some merely whispering was an enormous and taxing challenge—it was hard to get them to stop the flow of feelings they'd been forced to repress. They did not waste time with small talk. Most said they had learned about their illnesses not from their doctors but from a change in the behavior of their family and friends. Suddenly there was a distance and a dishonesty when what they desperately needed was the truth. Most of them felt their nurses were more empathic and helpful than their doctors. "Now's your chance to tell them why," I said.

I've always said the dying were my best teachers, but it took courage to listen to them. Patients weren't shy about expressing their dissatisfaction with their medical care—not the actual

147

physical care but the lack of compassion, empathy and understanding. Experienced doctors found it difficult to hear themselves painted as insensitive, frightened and inadequate. I remember one woman literally crying out, "All my doctor wants to discuss is the size of my liver. At this point, what do I care about the size of my liver? I have five children at home who need to be taken care of. That's what's killing me. And no one will talk to me about that!"

At the end of these interviews, patients felt relief. Many who had given up hope and felt useless reveled in their new role as teacher. Although they were dying, they realized it was possible for their lives to still have purpose, that they had a reason to live right till the final breath. They were still growing, and so were those in the audience.

After each interview, I took the patient back to his room and then returned to the lecture hall for lively, emotionally charged discussions. In addition to analyzing the patient's responses, we examined our own reactions. The admissions could be, and usually were, startling in their frankness. "I can hardly recall seeing a dead person," said one doctor about a fear of death that caused her to avoid it completely. "I don't know what to say," admitted a priest in reference to what he found were the Bible's limitations in answering the questions patients asked. "So I don't say anything."

In these discussions, doctors, priests and social workers confronted their hostility and defensiveness. Their fears were analyzed and overcome. By listening to dying patients, all of us learned what we should've done differently in the past and what we could do better in the future.

Each time I brought a patient in and then took him out, his life reminded me of "one of the millions of lights in a vast sky that flares up for a brief moment only to disappear into the endless night." The lessons each individual taught us boiled down to the same message:

Live so that you don't look back and regret that you've wasted your life.

Live so you don't regret the things you have done or wish that you had acted differently.

Live life honestly and fully.

Live.

CHAPTER TWENTY

Heart and Soul

❧

In my constant search for patients I could use in my Friday seminars, I developed a ritual of stalking the hospital corridors at night before I went home. Few of my colleagues wanted to help me. At home, Manny could listen to my frustrated rantings only up to a point before losing patience. He had his own work. Often I felt like the loneliest one in the whole hospital, so lonely that one night I walked into the chaplain's office.

I had no idea what a favor I did myself. The hospital's chaplain, the Reverend Renford Gaines, was at his desk. He was a tall, handsome black man in his mid-thirties. His movements, like his words, were slow and thoughtful. I knew the Reverend Gaines well from my seminars. He attended regularly and was one of my more interested students. Not surprisingly, he found that the discussions and insights he got there helped him counsel dying patients and their families.

That night the Reverend Gaines and I were on the same wavelength. We agreed that talking about death and dying taught us that the real questions most dying patients had concerned life, not death. They wanted honesty, closure and peace. It underscored that how a person died depended on how he lived. This included both the practical and the philosophical realms, the psychological and the spiritual—in other words, the two worlds that both of us occupied.

Over the next few weeks, the two of us spent hours locked in conversation, which usually prevented me from getting home and fixing dinner at a reasonable hour. But we inspired and taught each other. For someone like me who was schooled in the reason of science, the Reverend Gaines's world of the spirit was intellectual food I gobbled up. Ordinarily I avoided issues of spirituality in my seminars and talks with patients, since I was a psychiatrist. But the Reverend Gaines's interest in my work presented a unique opportunity. With his background, I could expand the reach of my work to include religion.

During one of our discussions, I asked my newfound friend and ally to serve as my partner. Thankfully, he accepted. From then on, the Reverend Gaines accompanied me when I visited terminally ill patients and assisted me during the seminars. Stylistically, we complemented each other perfectly. I asked what was going on inside a patient's head. The Reverend Gaines inquired about his soul. Our back-and-forth had the rhythm of a good Ping-Pong game. The seminars grew even more meaningful.

Others thought so too. The most important of these were the patients themselves. Only one out of two hundred refused to discuss the problems resulting from their illness. You perhaps wonder why they were so willing, but consider the first patient the Reverend Gaines and I presented together. Mrs. G., a middle-aged woman, had suffered from cancer for months, and during her hospitalization she made sure everyone from family members to nurses suffered along with her. But after several weeks of counseling, the Reverend Gaines soothed her anger and mended her relationships so that she was talking, really talking, and enjoying the people she loved. And they loved her back.

By the time of our seminar, Mrs. G. was a frail shell but also utterly transformed. "I've never lived so much in my entire adult life," she admitted.

The most unexpected vote of confidence came in early 1969. After more than three years of conducting my seminars, I received a delegation from the nearby Lutheran Seminary of Chicago. I anticipated a heated debate. Instead they asked me to join their faculty. Not surprisingly, I attempted to argue myself out of contention by presenting all kinds of excuses why they did not want me, including my dislike of religion. But they insisted. "We are not asking you to teach theology," they explained. "We are quite good at that. But we believe you can show us what real ministry means in practical terms."

It was hard to dispute them, since I agreed it was a good idea to have a teacher who spoke in nontheological language about ministering to dying patients. Except for the Reverend Gaines and the theology students, my experience with ministers had been dismal. Over the years most of the patients who had asked to speak to hospital chaplains had been disappointed. "All they want to do is read from their little black book," I heard repeatedly. In effect, real questions had been sidestepped in place of some convenient quotation from the Bible and a quick exit by a chaplain who was unsure of what to do.

That caused more harm than good. I can illustrate this with a story about a twelve-year-old girl named Liz. I met her several years after I'd been at the Seminary, but it is still relevant to the point. Dying of cancer, she was taken home, where I helped her mother, father and three brothers and sisters work through their various difficulties with her slow deterioration. But at the end, this little girl, who had withered to a skeleton with a huge, tumor-filled belly, knew the facts of her condition but refused to die anyway. "How come you can't die?" I asked her.

"Because I can't get to heaven," she said tearfully. "The priests and the sisters told me that no one gets to heaven unless they love God more than anybody else in the whole world." More sniffles. Then Liz pulled herself closer to me. "Dr. Ross, I love my mommy and daddy more than anybody else in the whole world."

On the verge of tears myself, I spoke symbolically about how God had given this very tough assignment to her. It was the same as when her teachers gave the hardest problems only to the very top students. She understood and said, "I don't think God could give a tougher assignment to any child."

It helped, and a few days later Liz was finally able to let go. But that was the type of case that soured me on religion.

Still the Lutherans persuaded me to accept the teaching job. My first lecture, only two weeks after the meeting, was in front of a packed auditorium. No one had any questions about how I felt about religion, particularly when I opened by questioning their concept of sin. "Besides promoting guilt and fear, what good is it?

151

"It does nothing more constructive than supply psychiatrists with business!" I added with a laugh to let them know I was also playing devil's advocate.

In subsequent classes, I tried to provoke them into examining their commitment to a life as a minister. If they thought it was difficult debating why the world needed different, often conflicting religious denominations when all of them attempted to teach the same basic wisdom, they were going to find the future pretty tough.

I became so popular that the seminary asked if I would screen prospective students and weed out ones who were not going to make it. That was interesting. About one-third of the students I spoke with ended up leaving the seminary. Instead they became social workers or entered related fields. On the whole, the experience of lecturing and interviewing students was fascinating. But I left after one semester. The demands on my busy schedule were too much for even a workaholic like me.

I already had the most interesting lecture job. I was never surprised at how much a dying patient could teach in one of my seminars, nor was I ever surprised at what the students taught themselves. I often felt wrong in taking credit for anything. In fact, my biggest nightmare was being stuck onstage alone for ten minutes without a patient. Just the thought of it made me panic. What would I say?

Then one day it happened. Ten minutes before a seminar was to begin, the patient I planned to interview unexpectedly died. With about eighty people seated in the auditorium, some of whom had traveled quite a distance to the hospital, I didn't want to cancel. On the other hand, there was no way I could find a substitute patient. Frozen in the hallway, where I could hear students buzzing inside the auditorium, I had no idea what to do without the one person I always presented as the real teacher.

But once I got onstage, I let inspiration take over and the class turned out to be fantastic. Since the majority of the audience worked in or were connected to the hospital/medical school, I asked what the biggest problem was in their daily work. Instead of talking to a patient, we'd discuss their biggest challenge. "Tell me what gives you the most difficulty," I said.

At first, the room was perfectly silent, but after a few uneasy moments several hands went up. Much to my surprise the first two people called on said that one particular physician, actually a department head, who worked almost exclusively with very sick cancer patients, was a problem. He was brilliant, they explained, but if anyone even hinted that one of his patients might not respond to treatment, the doctor snapped back in a nasty tone. Others in the audience, knowing this person, nodded in agreement.

Although I didn't say anything, I immediately recognized the doctor from my own numerous run-ins with him. I couldn't stand his abrupt manner, his arrogance or his dishonesty. On two occasions in my capacity as head of the psychosomatic liaison service, I'd been called in to consult with his dying patients. He'd told one that he was free of cancer and another that it was only a matter of time before she'd feel better. Both of their X-rays showed large, inoperable metastases.

Clearly the doctor was the one who needed the shrink. He had a serious problem with death and dying, though I couldn't say that to either patient. I couldn't help them by criticizing someone else, especially someone they trusted.

But the seminar was different. We pretended that Dr. M. was the patient and talked about the problems we had with him. Then we discussed what these problems told us about ourselves. Almost the entire audience admitted to having a bias against colleagues, their fellow doctors and nurses, who had troubles. They judged them differently than they did normal patients. I agreed and used my own feelings toward Dr. M. as an example. "You can't help another human unless you like them a little bit," I said.

But then I raised a question: "Is there anybody here who likes him?"

Amid many hostile looks and sneers, a young woman slowly, hesitantly raised her hand into the air. "Are you sick?" I asked, half in jest, half amazed. A good laugh followed. Then this nurse stood, noble in her calm and clarity. "You don't know this man," she argued. "You don't know the person." There was now silence. Her fragile voice pierced the quiet with a detailed description of Dr. M. starting his rounds late at night, hours after other doctors had gone home.

"He starts in the room farthest away from the nursing station and makes his way toward where I usually sit," she explained. "He enters the first room standing straight, appearing confident and in control. But each time he leaves a room, his back is a little more bent. His posture looks more and more like that of an old man." The nurse reenacted the nightly drama, forcing everyone to picture the scene. "By the time he leaves the last patient's room, this doctor looks crushed. You can see that he's completely devoid of any joy, hope or satisfaction in his work."

Just watching this drama night after night affected her. Imagine the toll it took on the doctor! There wasn't a dry eye in the auditorium as the nurse confessed her long-standing desire to gently touch the doctor, as a friend would, and tell him she knew how hard and hopeless his job was. But the hospital's caste system prevented such human behavior. "I'm only a nurse," she said.

Yet this sort of compassion and friendly understanding was precisely the help that the doctor needed, and since this young nurse was the only one in the room who cared about him, she was the one who had to do it. I told her that she had to force herself to make a move. "Don't think about it," I said. "Just do whatever your heart tells you to do." Then I added, "If you help him, you'll help thousands and thousands of people."

After a week's vacation, I was catching up on work in my office when the door flew open and a young woman rushed in. She was the nurse from the previous seminar. "I did it!" she told me. "I did it!"

Starting that past Friday, she had watched Dr. M. make his rounds, ending up, as she had described, a broken man. The drama repeated itself on Saturday, but with a complication. Two of his patients had died that day. On Sunday she watched as he exited the last room, bent over and depressed. Forcing herself to act, she approached him, imploring herself to reach out. But before she could offer an arm, she exclaimed, "God, it must be so difficult!"

All of a sudden, Dr. M. grabbed her arm and pulled her into his office. Behind the closed door, she witnessed him releasing all of his pent-up pain, grief and anguish. He recounted all the sacrifices he made to make it through medical school; how his friends had jobs and incomes when he started his residency; and how he dreamed of making his patients well while his contemporaries were raising families and constructing vacation homes. His life had been about learning a specialty rather than living. Now, finally, he was chairman of his department. He had a position where he could really make a difference in the lives of his patients.

"But they all die," he sobbed. "One after another. They all die on me."

After hearing this story in the next Death and Dying seminar, everyone realized the extraordinary power a person has to heal just by summoning the courage to act from the heart. Within a year, Dr. M. began psychiatric consultations with me. About three years later, he was in therapy full time. His life improved dramatically. Instead of ending up a burned-out depressive, Dr. M. rediscovered the wonderful, caring and understanding qualities that had motivated him to become a doctor. If only he knew how many people my telling of his story has helped over the years.

CHAPTER TWENTY-ONE

My Mother

It should have felt perfect, the picture of contentment. In 1969, we moved into a beautiful home designed by Frank Lloyd Wright's firm, in Flossmoor, an upper-class suburb. My new garden sprawled over enough land so that Manny and the kids gave me a mini-tractor for my birthday. Manny loved his new study and installed a great stereo system so I could listen to country music while puttering in what was my dream kitchen. The children were enrolled in an outstanding public school.

But it struck me as almost too perfect to be right. It was like a dream that I expected to wake up from. Then one morning I did wake up knowing the source of my angst. Here we were in the land of plenty, where we wanted for nothing, except that I had not passed on to my children the thing that had been most important to my own childhood. I wanted them to know what it was like to get up early in the morning, hike in the hills and mountains, appreciate the flowers, the different grasses, the crickets and butterflies. I wanted them to gather wildflowers and colorful rocks during the day and then at night let the stars fill their heads with dreams.

I did not wait and ponder what I should do. That would not have been me. Acting swiftly, I took Kenneth and Barbara out of school the next week and flew home to Switzerland. My mother met us in Zermatt, a charming alpine village where automobiles were prohibited and life was pretty much as it was a hundred years before. That is what I wanted. The weather was heavenly. I took the children on hikes. They climbed mountains, ran along streams and chased animals. They picked flowers and brought home rocks. Their cheeks were sunburned. It was an unforgettable experience.

But, as it turned out, not because of that. On our final night, my mother and I put the children to bed. She lingered for some extra good-night kisses and hugs while I stepped out onto the balcony. I was rocking in an old hand-hewn chair when the sliding doors from the bedroom opened and she joined me in the fresh night air.

Both of us marveled at the moon. It seemed to be floating over the Matterhorn. My mother sat down beside me. We were silent for the longest time, thinking our thoughts. The week had been better than I had imagined. I could not have been happier. I thought of all the city dwellers in the world who never made the effort to see such a remarkable sky. They tolerated their lives by watching TV and drinking alcohol. My mother looked equally gratified, both in the moment and with her life.

I do not know how long we sat in silence, enjoying each other's company, but my mother finally cracked the spell. She could have said a million things at that moment, anything except what she did say: "Elisabeth, we don't live forever." There are reasons people do things at certain moments. I had no idea why my mother, at that time and in that setting, uttered such a thing. Maybe it was the enormity of the sky. Maybe it was that she felt relaxed and close after our week together.

Maybe, as I now believe, she had a premonition, a sense of the future.

In any event, she continued. "You are the only doctor in the family and if there is an emergency I will count on you."

What emergency? Despite being seventy-seven years old, she had managed every hike without complaint, without problem. She was perfectly healthy.

I did not know what to say. I wanted to shout something at her. But in reality, she did not leave me any space. She kept going in that morbid direction, saying, "If I ever become a vegetable, I want you to terminate my life." I listened with increasing annoyance and said something to the effect of "Stop talking like that," but my mother reiterated her statement. For whatever

158

reason, she was ruining the night and maybe the whole vacation. "Stop with such nonsense," I pleaded. "Nothing like that is going to happen."

My mother seemed not to care what I thought right then, and it was true that I could not ensure that she would not end up a vegetable. The whole conversation was very irritating. Finally I sat forward and told my mother that I was against suicide and would never—never ever—assist anyone, especially my mother, the loving person who gave birth to me and kept me alive. "If something happens, I will do the same for you that I do for all my patients," I said. "I will help you live until you die."

Somehow we found our way to the end of this disturbing conversation. There was no more to say. I got up from my chair and hugged my mother. Both of us had tears streaming down our cheeks. It was late, time for bed. The next day we were going to Zurich. I just wanted to think about the good times, not the future.

In the morning, the spell was broken. My mother was back to her old self and we enjoyed the train ride to Zurich. Manny met us in the city and we checked into a luxury hotel, which was more his style. I did not mind, since my "tank" was full of crisp alpine air and wildflowers. After one more week, we flew back to Chicago. I felt totally rejuvenated, except that I could not shake the talk I'd had with my mother. I tried not to pay attention, but it was a dark cloud on my conscience.

Then, three days later, Eva called me at home and told me that the mailman had found our mother lying on the bathroom floor. She had suffered a massive stroke.

I got on the next plane to Switzerland and went straight to my mother's hospital bed. Unable to move or speak, she stared at me with a hundred words in her deep, injured, pained and frightened eyes. They added up to one plea, which I understood. But I knew then—as I'd known before—that I could never fulfill her request. I could never be an instrument of her death.

The next few days were hard ones. I sat, waited and carried on a monologue with my mother. Though her body was unable to respond, she answered me with her eyes. One blink for yes. Two for no. At times, she was able to squeeze my hand with her left hand. By the end of the week, she suffered a few additional, smaller strokes. She lost control of her bladder. With that, she was considered a vegetable. "Are you comfortable?" One blink. "Do you want to stay here?" Two blinks.

"I love you."

She squeezed my hand.

It was exactly the condition she had feared during our vacation the previous week. She had even forewarned me. "If I ever become a vegetable, I want you to terminate my life." Her plea on the balcony echoed in my memory. Did she know this was coming? Did she have a premonition? Was such an inner awareness possible?

I asked myself, "How can I help her make this remaining time of her life more bearable? More enjoyable for her?"

So many questions. So few answers.

If there was a God, I mused silently, this was the time to enter her life, to thank her for selflessly loving her family, raising her children to become respectable, worthwhile, productive human beings. At night, I had long conversations with Him. One afternoon I even entered a church and spoke directly to the cross. "God, where are You?" I asked bitterly. "Can You hear me at all? Do You even exist? My mother was a clean, dedicated, hardworking woman. What do You plan on doing for her now that she really needs You?" But there was no answer. No sign.

Nothing but silence.

Watching my mother languish in her cocoon of helplessness and torment, I almost screamed out loud for some heavenly interference. Privately, I commanded God to do something, and do it fast. But if God heard me, He didn't seem to be in a hurry. I called Him nasty names in Swiss and English. He still wasn't impressed.

Although we had lengthy discussions with hospital doctors and outside consultants, we were left with two choices. Either my mother could remain in this teaching hospital, where every procedure would be tried, though chances for even the smallest recovery were slim. Or we could move her to a less expensive rest home where she would get good nursing care but no artificial efforts would be made to prolong her life. In other words, no respirators or machines.

160

My sisters and I had a long, emotional conversation. All three of us knew what our mother would have chosen. Manny, who considered my mother to be a second mother, offered his expert opinion via long-distance. Thankfully, Eva had already located an excellent nursing home run by Protestant nuns in Riehen, near Basel, where she and her new husband had built a new house. This was in the days before hospices, but the nuns dedicated their lives to caring for such special patients. Mustering all of our influence, we got my mother admitted.

With my time off from the hospital running out, I decided to accompany my mother in the ambulance from Zurich to Riehen. To give us both courage, I brought along a large bottle of *Eiercognac*—spiced eggnog with cognac. I also made a list, which was rather short, of my mother's most beloved possessions, and also a list of relatives and significant people in her life, especially those who'd helped her in the years after my father died. That was a longer one.

During the drive, we distributed her things to the proper individuals. It took a long time to figure out who got what, like the mink collar and hat we had sent from New York. But whenever I matched a person to the right item, we celebrated with a sip of the cognac-and-eggnog drink. The ambulance attendant seemed a little unsure about that, but I said, "It's okay, I'm a doctor."

Not only did we accomplish something that would give my mother peace of mind; by the time we reached the nursing home we were actually enjoying ourselves. My mother's room looked out onto a garden. She settled in well. During the day, she would be able to hear birds singing in the trees. At night, she would have a view of the sky. Before I said goodbye, I tucked a perfumed handkerchief into her one semi-good hand. Ordinarily she held one like that. I saw she was relaxed and content, in a place where she knew the quality of her life was the top consideration.

For some reason, God saw fit to keep her alive like this for four more years. Her condition defied all the odds of survival. My sisters made sure that she was perfectly comfortable and never lonely. I visited frequently. Always my thoughts went back to that fateful night in Zermatt. I heard her begging me to terminate her life if she ended up a vegetable. She obviously had a premonition, because now she embodied the very picture she had feared. It was tragic.

Still, I knew it was not the end. My mother continued to feel love and give love. In her own way, she was growing and learning whatever lessons she needed to learn. Everybody should know that. Life ends when you have learned everything you are supposed to learn. Therefore any thought of ending her life, as she had asked, was even more unimaginable than before.

I wanted to know why my mother ended up like this. I constantly asked myself what lesson God was trying to teach this loving woman.

I even wondered if she was teaching the rest of us a lesson.

But as long as she continued to survive without artificial life support, there was nothing to do, except to love her.

The Purpose of Life

❦

It was inevitable that I had to look beyond the hospital. My work with dying patients made a lot of my colleagues very uneasy. Few people at the hospital wanted to talk about death. It was even hard to find someone who would admit that people there were dying. Death just was not something that doctors talked about. So when my weekly search for dying patients became nearly impossible, I began making house calls on cancer patients in surrounding neighborhoods like Homewood and Flossmoor.

I offered a mutually beneficial deal. In exchange for free bedside therapy, patients agreed to be interviewed at my seminars. This approach stirred up more controversy around the hospital, where my work was already called exploitative. Then it got worse. As patients and their families spoke publicly about how much they appreciated my work, the other doctors found another reason to resent me. I could not win.

But I behaved like a winner. On top of motherhood and work, I volunteered with several organizations. Once a month I screened candidates for the Peace Corps. They probably had mixed feelings about me, since I tended to approve all those considered to be risk takers, not the middle-of-the-roaders my associates preferred. I also spent a half day each week at Chicago's Lighthouse for the Blind, working with parents and children. But I have a feeling they gave more back to me.

The people I met there, adults and children alike, were all

struggling with the bad hands they had been dealt by fate. I studied how they coped. Their lives were a roller coaster of misery and courage, depression and accomplishment. I constantly asked myself what I, as a sighted person, could do to help. Mainly I listened, but I was also a cheerleader, encouraging them to "see" it was still possible for them to live full, productive and happy lives. Life was a challenge, not a tragedy.

Sometimes that was a lot to ask. I saw far too many babies born blind, as well as others born with hydrocephalus, who were written off as vegetables and placed in institutions for the rest of their lives. Such a waste of life. So were those parents who did not find help or support. I noticed that so many parents who gave birth to blind children went through the same reactions as my dying patients. Reality was often difficult to accept. But what was the choice?

I recall one mother who had gone through nine months of a normal pregnancy with no reason to expect anything but a normal, healthy child. But in the delivery room, something happened and her daughter was born blind. She reacted as though there had been a death in the family, which was normal. But after being helped through the initial trauma, she began hoping that her daughter, named Heidi, would one day graduate from school and learn a profession. That was healthy and wonderful.

Unfortunately, she got involved with some professionals who said her dreams were unrealistic. They encouraged her to put the baby in an institution. The family was heartbroken. But thankfully, before taking any steps, they sought help at the Lighthouse, which was how I met this woman.

Obviously I could not offer any miracles that would return her daughter's eyesight, but I did listen to her troubles. And then when she asked what I thought, I told this mother, who wanted so badly to find a miracle, that no child was born so defective that God did not endow him with a special gift. "Drop all your expectations," I said. "All you have to do is hold and love your child like she was a gift from God."

"And then?" she asked.

"In time, He will reveal her special gift," I replied.

I had no idea where those words of mine came from, but I believed them. And the mother left with renewed hope.

Many years later, I was reading a newspaper when I noticed an article about Heidi, the little girl from the Lighthouse. All grown up, Heidi was a promising pianist and was performing in public for the first time. The local critic raved about her talent. I wasted no time looking up her mother, who proudly told me how she had struggled to raise her daughter. Then all of a sudden, Heidi developed a gift for music. It just blossomed, like a flower, and her mother credited my encouraging words.

"It would have been so easy to reject her," she said. "That's what the other people told me to do."

Naturally I shared these kinds of rewarding moments with my family and hoped they learned not to take anything for granted. There were no guarantees in life, except that everyone faces struggles. It is how we learn. Some face struggle from the moment they are born. They are the most special of all people, requiring the most care and compassion and reminding us that love is the sole purpose of life.

Believe it or not, there were some people who actually thought I knew what I was talking about. One such person was Clement Alexander, an editor at the Macmillan publishing house in New York. Somehow a short paper I had written about my Death and Dying seminars landed on his desk. That caused him to fly out to Chicago and ask if I wanted to write a book about my work with dying patients. I was dumbstruck, even as he gave me a contract to sign, offering $7,000 in exchange for 50,000 words.

Well, I agreed, so long as I had three months in which to write the book. That was not a problem for Macmillan. But then I was left by myself to figure out how I was planning to manage two children, a husband, a full-time job and various other things, plus writing a book. I noticed the contract already had given my book a title, *On Death and Dying*. I liked it. I called Manny and told him the good news. Then I began to think of myself as an author and I could not believe it.

But why not? I had countless case histories and observations piled up in my head. It took three weeks of sitting at my desk late at night, while Kenneth and Barbara slept, before I figured out the book. Then I saw very clearly how all of my dying patients, in fact everyone who suffers a loss, went through similar stages.

They started off with shock and denial, rage and anger, and then grief and pain. Later they bargained with God. They got depressed, asking, "Why me?" And finally they withdrew into themselves for a bit, separating themselves from others while hopefully reaching a stage of peace and acceptance (not resignation, which occurs when tears and anger are not shared).

I actually saw these stages most clearly in the parents I had met at the Lighthouse. They associated the birth of a blind child with loss—the loss of the normal and healthy child they expected. They went through shock and anger, denial and depression, and with some therapy finally managed to accept what could not be changed.

People who had lost or were in the process of losing a next of kin went through the same five stages, starting with denial and shock. "It can't possibly be that my wife is dying. She just had a baby. How can she leave me?" Or they exclaimed, "No, not me, I can't be dying." Denial is a defense, a normal, healthy way of coping with horrible, unexpected, sudden bad news. It allows a person to consider the possible end of her life and then return to life as it's always been.

When denial is no longer feasible it's replaced by anger. Rather than continue to ask, "Why me?" the patient asks, "Why not him?" This stage is especially difficult for families, doctors, nurses, friends etc. The patient's anger scatters like buckshot. Fragments fly in every direction. It hits everyone. He rages at God, his family, at anyone who is healthy. The patient might as well be screaming, "I'm alive and don't you forget that." His anger shouldn't be taken personally.

If patients were allowed to express their anger without guilt or shame, they often went through a stage of bargaining. "Oh, please let my wife live long enough to see this child enter kindergarten." Then they added a quickie prayer. "Wait at least until she finishes high school. Then she'll be old enough to cope with the death of her mother." And so on. Pretty soon I noticed the promises people made to God were never kept. They literally bargained, raising the ante each time.

But the time spent bargaining is beneficial for the caregivers. The patient, although angry, is no longer so consumed by hostility that he can't hear. The patient is not depressed to the point where he can't communicate anymore. They may be firing bullets, but they're not hitting anything. I advised that this was the best time to help patients complete whatever unfinished business they had. Go into their rooms. Confront old squabbles. Add fuel to the fire. Let them externalize their anger, let go of it, and then the old hatreds will turn into love and understanding.

At some point, patients will find themselves severely depressed over the huge changes taking place. Naturally. Who wouldn't? Either their illness can no longer be denied or severe physical limitations set in. Over time there might also be financial burdens. There are often drastic, debilitating changes in appearance. A woman worries that the loss of a breast makes her less of a woman. When concerns like these are openly, forthrightly addressed, patients often respond beautifully.

The more difficult type of depression results from a patient's realization that he is going to lose everything and everyone he loves. It's a kind of silent depression. In this state, there is no bright side. Nor are there any soothing words that can be said to alleviate the state of mind that's given up on the past and is trying to fathom the unfathomable future. The best help is to allow the patient his sorrow, say a prayer, simply give him a loving touch or just sit with him on the bed.

If patients have been allowed to express their anger, to cry and grieve, to finish their unfinished business, to articulate their fears, to work through the above stages, they will reach the last stage of acceptance. They won't be happy, but they will no longer be depressed or angry. It's a period of quiet, meditative resignation, of peaceful expectancy. The previous struggle disappears and is replaced by the need for lots of sleep, which, in *On Death and Dying*, I described a patient calling "the final rest before the long journey."

After two months, I finished the book. I realized that I had created exactly the kind of book I had hoped to find in the library when I went to research my first lecture. I dropped the final draft in the mailbox. Although I had no idea whether *On Death and Dying* would become an important book, I was absolutely sure the information I had set down was very important. I hoped people would not misconstrue the message. My dying patients never healed in the physical sense, but they all got better emotionally and spiritually. In fact, they felt a lot better than most healthy people.

Later someone would ask what all those dying patients had taught me about death. First I thought about giving them a very clinical explanation, but then I would have misrepresented myself. My dying patients taught me so much more than what it was like to be dying. They shared lessons about what they could have done, and what they should have done, and what they didn't do until it was too late, until they were too sick or too weak, until they were widowers or widows. They looked back at their lives and taught me all of the things that were really meaningful, not about dying . . . but about living.

CHAPTER TWENTY-THREE

Fame

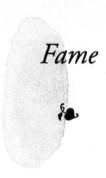

It was a bad day at work. One of my residents, somewhat reluctantly, asked if I had time to advise him on a problem. Thinking it was something to do with his relationship, I said okay. But then he said that he had been offered a position in my own department at a starting salary of $15,000. He wanted to know if that was acceptable.

Since I was his superior, I tried to hide my shock and disbelief. My own salary was $3,000 less. It was not the first time I had experienced a bias against women, but that did not make me any less disgusted.

Then the Reverend Gaines told me that he was going to look for a new position. Tired of all the hospital politics, he wanted his own parish, a place where he could try to effect real change in the community. I got depressed thinking about not having the daily support of my only true ally at the hospital.

I went home, wanting to stand in the kitchen and disappear from the world. But even that was impossible. I got a call from a *Life* magazine reporter. He asked if he could write a story on my Death and Dying seminar at the university. I took a deep breath, a good thing to do when you do not know what to say. Although naive about publicity, I was tired of not having any support. I said yes, sensing that if my work was better known it could actually change the quality of countless lives.

Once the reporter and I agreed on an interview date, I set about finding a patient for the seminar. It was harder than normal, since the Reverend Gaines happened to be out of town. His boss, having heard about the *Life* article, ambitiously substituted himself, but he was no help in finding me a dying patient to interview.

Then one dreary day, as I walked down the I-3 hallway, the ward occupied by most of the cancer patients, I glanced through a half-open door. At that moment, my thoughts were elsewhere. I was not even thinking about finding a patient. But I was struck by the unusually pretty girl in that room. I am sure I was not the first person who had ever looked at her and stopped.

But her eyes also caught mine and drew me into the room. Her name was Eva. She was twenty-one years old. She was a dark-haired beauty, pretty enough to have become an actress, if she had not been dying of leukemia. But she was still a real pistol, outgoing, funny, dreamy and warm. She was also engaged. "See," she said, showing me her ring. Life should have been ahead of her.

Instead she talked about her life as it was right then. She wanted her body donated to a medical school, not a funeral. She was angry at her fiancé for not accepting her illness. "He's wasting our time," she said. "After all, I don't have much longer." What I realized, quite happily, was that Eva wanted to live as much as possible, still have experiences that were new, including attending one of my seminars. She had heard of them and asked if she could participate. It was the first time a dying patient had beaten me to the queston.

"Doesn't my leukemia make me eligible?" she asked.

There was no doubt, but first I wanted to warn her about *Life* magazine.

"Yes!" she exclaimed. "I want to do it."

I suggested that she might want to talk it over with her parents.

"I don't have to," she said. "I'm twenty-one years old. I can make my own decisions."

She certainly could, and at the end of the week I wheeled her down the hall toward my classroom. There we were, two females worrying about how our hair was going to look for the camera. Once we got in front of the students, my hunch about Eva was proved correct. She was an extraordinary subject.

First of all, Eva was about the same age as most of the

170

students, which made the point that death does not take only the old. She also looked striking. In a white blouse and tweed slacks, she could have been going out to a cocktail party. But she was dying, and her frankness about that reality was the most stunning thing about her. "I know my chances are one in a million," she confessed. "But today I only wish to talk about this one chance."

So instead of talking about her illness, Eva spoke about what it would be like if she could live. Her thoughts spanned school, marriage and children, her family and God. "When I was little, I used to believe in God," she said. "Now I don't know." Eva explained that she wanted a puppy and to go home once more. She exposed her raw emotions without hesitation. Neither of us thought once about the reporter or the photographer who were chronicling everything we said and did on our side of the two-way mirror, but we knew it was good.

The magazine article came out November 21, 1969. My telephone began ringing before I even saw the issue. But my concern was Eva's reaction. That night several copies of the magazine were delivered to me at home. Early the next morning I raced to the hospital to show them to Eva before they hit the hospital newsstand and made her an instant celebrity. Thankfully, Eva approved of the article, but like any healthy, normal, pretty woman, she shook her head disapprovingly at the photos. "Gosh, they aren't very good of me," she said.

The hospital was not as pleased as we were. The first doctor I saw in the hallway sneered and in a nasty tone asked, "Looking for another patient for publicity?" One administrator criticized me for making the hospital famous for dying. "Our reputation is for making people better," he said. For most, the *Life* article was proof I exploited my patients. They did not get it. A week later the hospital took measures to thwart my seminars by ordering doctors not to cooperate with me. It was terrible. On the next Friday, I faced a virtually empty auditorium.

Although humiliated, I knew they could not undo everything that had been put into motion by the press. There I was, in one of the country's biggest, most respected magazines. Mail piled up for me in the hospital's mailroom. The switchboard was flooded with callers wanting to know how to get in touch with me. I did more interviews and even agreed to speak at other universities and colleges.

There was more attention with the release of my book, *On Death and Dying*. It was an international best-seller and virtually every nursing and medical institution in the country recognized it as an important book. Even ordinary people found themselves discussing the five stages. Little did I suspect that the book would be so successful or prove to be my entry into the world of fame. Ironically, the only place where it did not enjoy instant acceptance was the psychiatric unit of my own hospital, a clear indication that my future would be spent elsewhere.

In the meantime, my main interest never veered from my patients, who were the real teachers. This was especially true with my *Life* magazine girl, Eva. I was particularly concerned when I poked my head into her room on New Year's Eve and did not see her there. I breathed a sigh of relief when someone said she had gone home and gotten the puppy she had wanted. But it also turned out that she had then been transferred to the Intensive Care Unit. I hurried over there and saw her parents in the waiting-room area.

They had that sad, helpless look I saw so often in the families of dying patients as they sat in waiting rooms, prevented by stupid visiting-hour rules from being with their loved ones. Per the ICU rules, Eva's parents were allowed to see her for only five minutes at appointed hours. I was outraged. This might be the last day they could sit with their daughter, supporting and loving each other. What if she died while they were seated outside her room?

As a doctor, I was allowed in Eva's room, and when I entered I found her lying naked on top of her bed. The overhead light, which she could not control, was on constantly, casting a bright glare on her from which she had no means of escape. I knew this was going to be the last time I saw her alive. So did Eva. Unable to speak, she pressed my hand as a way of saying hello and pointed her other hand up toward the ceiling. She wanted the light off.

Her comfort and dignity were all that mattered to me. I turned off the light and then asked a nurse to cover Eva with a bedsheet. Unbelievably the nurse hesitated. She felt as if I were wasting her time. She asked, "Why?" Why cover this girl? I was furious and did it myself.

Sadly, Eva died the next day, January 1, 1970. I had no control over her life, but the way she had died in the hospital, cold and alone, was something I could not tolerate. All my work was aimed at changing that kind of situation. I did not want anyone to die like Eva, by herself, with her family waiting outside in the hall. I dreamed of the day when the needs of a human being would come first.

CHAPTER TWENTY-FOUR

Mrs. Schwartz

Everything changed with the miraculous new advances in medicine. Doctors extended lives with heart and kidney transplants and powerful new drugs. New equipment helped diagnose trouble earlier. Patients whose problems would have been incurable a year earlier were being given second chances at life. It was exciting. Still, there were problems. People were deluded into believing medicine could fix everything. There were previously unforeseen ethical, moral, legal and financial issues. And I saw doctors making decisions in consultation with insurance companies, not other physicians.

"It's only going to get worse," I said to the Reverend Gaines. But it did not take a genius to make that prediction. Already the writing was on the wall. The hospital had been slapped with several lawsuits, something that was happening more frequently than I ever recalled. But medicine was changing. The ethics seemed to be undergoing a rewrite. "I wish it was the way it used to be," said the Reverend Gaines. My solution was different. "The real problem is that we don't have a true definition of death," I said.

From the time of the cavemen, no one had come up with an exact definition of death. I was wondering what happened to my beautiful patients, people like Eva, who shared so much one day and then were gone the next. Soon the Reverend Gaines and I were asking groups that included medical and theology students, plus doctors, rabbis and priests, where life went. "If not here, then where?" I was trying to define death.

175

I opened myself up to every possibility, even some of the silly notions my children proposed at the dinner table. I never hid my work from them, which helped all of us. Looking at Kenneth and Barbara, I concluded that birth and death were similar experiences—each the start of a new journey. But later I would conclude that death was the more pleasant of the two, much more peaceful. Our world was full of Nazis, AIDS, cancer and stuff like that.

I noticed how patients, even the angriest of them, relaxed moments before death. Others appeared to have extremely vivid experiences with deceased loved ones as they neared death themselves, talking with people I could not see. In virtually every case, death was preceded by a peculiar serenity.

And then? That was the question I wanted to answer.

I could only make judgments based on my observations. And once they died, I felt nothing. They were gone. One day I could talk and touch someone and the next morning they were not there. Their body was, but that was like touching a piece of wood. Something was missing. Something physical. Life itself.

"But in what form did life leave?" I continued to ask. "And where, if anywhere, did it go? What did people experience at the moment they died?"

At some point my thoughts returned to my trip to Maidanek twenty-five years earlier. Back then I had walked through the barracks where men, women and children had spent their final nights before dying in the gas chamber. I remembered being spellbound by the sight of butterflies drawn on the walls and wondering: Why butterflies . . . ?

Now, in a flash of clarity, I knew. Those prisoners were like my dying patients and aware of what was going to happen. They knew that soon they would become butterflies. Once dead, they would be out of that hellish place. Not tortured anymore. Not separated from their families. Not sent to gas chambers. None of this gruesome life mattered anymore. Soon they would leave their bodies the way a butterfly leaves its cocoon. And I realized that was the message they wanted to leave for future generations.

It also provided the imagery that I would use for the rest of my career to explain the process of death and dying. But I still wanted to know more. One day I turned to my minister partner and said,

176

"You guys are always saying, 'Ask and you will be given.' Okay, now I'm asking. Help me do research on death." He did not have a ready answer, but both of us believed that the right question usually got a good answer.

A week later, a nurse told me about a woman who she thought might make a good interview candidate. Mrs. Schwartz had been in and out of the ICU more than a dozen times. Each time she had been expected to die. Each time this amazingly resilient, determined woman had survived. The nurses looked at her with a mix of awe and respect. "I think she's also a little strange," the nurse told me. "She frightens me."

There was nothing frightening about Mrs. Schwartz when I interviewed her for the Death and Dying seminar. She explained that her husband was a schizophrenic who attacked their youngest child, a seventeen-year-old boy, each time he had a psychotic episode. She feared that if she died before her son came of age, his life would be endangered. With her husband as the sole legal guardian, there was no telling what might happen when he lost control. "That's why I can't die yet," she explained.

Acknowledging her real concerns, I brought in a lawyer from the Legal Aid Society, who helped transfer custody of the child to a healthier, more reliable relative. Relieved, Mrs. Schwartz left the hospital once more, grateful she could live whatever time remained in peace. I didn't expect to see her again.

Not quite a year later, though, she knocked at my office door, pleading to return to my seminar. I said no. My policy was not to repeat cases. Students had to be able to speak with total strangers about the most taboo subjects. "But that's why I need to talk to them," she said. After a long pause, she added, "And to you."

A week later, I reluctantly ushered Mrs. Schwartz in front of a new group of students. At first, she told the same story that I heard before. Fortunately, most of the students hadn't. Disappointed in myself for letting her return, I interrupted her and asked, "What was so urgent that you had to come back to my seminar?" That was all the prompting she needed. Switching gears, Mrs. Schwartz recounted what turned out to be the first near-death experience any of us had heard, though we didn't call it that.

The incident happened in Indiana. Felled by internal bleeding,

Mrs. Schwartz was rushed to a hospital and put in a private room, where her condition was pronounced "critical" and too dire for her to be sent back to Chicago. Feeling that she was close to death this time, she debated whether or not to call for a nurse. She asked herself how many more times she wanted to go through this life-and-death ordeal. Now that her son was taken care of, perhaps she was ready to die.

She was very blunt. Part of her wanted to let go. But another part of her wanted to survive till her son came of age.

As she debated what to do, a nurse entered the room, took one look at her and dashed out without saying a word. According to Mrs. Schwartz, at precisely that moment she floated out of her physical body and toward the ceiling. Then a resuscitation team raced in the room and worked frantically to save her.

All the while Mrs. Schwartz watched from above the room. She took in every bit of detail. She heard what everyone said. She even sensed what they were thinking. Remarkably, she had no pain, fear or anxiety about being out of her body. Just enormous curiosity and wonderment that they did not listen to her. She repeatedly asked them to stop the heroics and assured them she was okay. "But they did not hear," she said.

She finally went down and poked one of the residents, but to her amazement, her arm went right through his arm. At that point, as frustrated as her doctors, Mrs. Schwartz described giving up on them. "Then I lost consciousness," she explained. After forty-five minutes, Mrs. Schwartz's last observation was of them covering her with a bedsheet and pronouncing her dead, while an anxious and defeated resident told jokes. But three and a half hours later a nurse came into the room to remove her body and instead found Mrs. Schwartz alive.

Her amazing story captivated everyone in the auditorium. People instantly turned to the person next to them and began trying to decide whether or not they should believe whatever it was they had just heard. After all, most of the people in the room were scientists. They wondered if she was crazy. Mrs. Schwartz had the same question. When I asked why she was willing to tell us this experience, she asked, "Am I psychotic now, too?"

No, certainly not. By then I knew Mrs. Schwartz well enough to know she was very sane and telling the truth. Yet Mrs. Schwartz was not so sure and needed confirmation. Before leaving, she again asked, "Do you think I was psychotic?" She sounded distressed, while I was in a hurry to wrap up the session. So I responded declaring, "I, Dr. Elisabeth Kübler-Ross, can verify that you are not now and never have been psychotic."

With that, Mrs. Schwartz finally leaned back on her pillow and relaxed. Right then I knew she wasn't crazy at all. That woman had all her marbles intact.

* * *

In the discussion that followed, students wanted to know why I had pretended to believe Mrs. Schwartz, instead of admitting she had hallucinated the whole thing. Surprisingly, I don't think there was a person in the room who believed that what Mrs. Schwartz experienced was real, that at the moment of death human beings maintain an awareness, that they can still make observations, have thoughts, not suffer pain, and that it has nothing to do with psychopathology.

"Then what do you call it?" another student asked.

I did not have a quick answer, which angered my students, but I explained there were still many things we did not know or understand, which did not negate their existence. "If I blew a dog whistle right now, none of us would hear it," I said. "But every dog would. Does that mean it doesn't exist?" Was it possible that Mrs. Schwartz had been on a different wavelength than the rest of us? "How could she have repeated a joke one of the doctors had told? Explain that." Just because we weren't able to see what she had, did that discount the reality of her vision?

Hard answers were going to have to come in the future. But then I wrapped up by explaining that Mrs. Schwartz had a motive for appearing at the seminar. After no students were able to guess it, I explained that it was purely a motherly concern. Also, Mrs. Schwartz knew the seminar was tape-recorded and contained eighty witnesses. "If her episode had been labeled psychotic, then the legal arrangements for her son's custody could have been voided," I said. "Her husband could've then gained control of their child and destroyed her peace of mind. Was she crazy? Absolutely not."

Mrs. Schwartz's story haunted me for weeks afterward, since I knew what happened to her could not be a unique experience. If one person who had died was able to recall something as extraordinary as a team of doctors trying to bring her back after her vital signs had stopped, then others probably could too. Suddenly the Reverend Gaines and I turned into detectives. Our intention was to interview twenty individuals who had been revived after their vital signs indicated they had died. If my hunch was right, we would soon be opening the door to a brand-new facet of the human condition, a whole new awareness of life.

CHAPTER TWENTY-FIVE

Afterlife

A s investigators, the Reverend Gaines and I kept our distance. No, it was not because we had a misunderstanding. Rather it was that we agreed not to compare notes until we each had twenty cases. We combed the hallways alone. We utilized outside resources. We made inquiries and followed up leads in search of patients who fit our criteria. We never had to ask a patient to do more than tell us what happened or what he felt. They were so anxious to have somebody interested in listening that stories just poured out.

And when the Reverend Gaines and I finally compared notes, we were astounded, as well as thrilled beyond description, by the material we had collected. "Yes, I saw my father clear as day," one patient confessed to me. Another person thanked the Reverend Gaines for asking. "I'm so glad I can talk with someone about that. Everybody I've told has treated me like I was crazy, and it was so beautiful and peaceful." We kept going. "I could see again," said a woman who had been blinded in an accident. But once she was brought back to the world, her sight left her again.

This was long before anyone had written about near-death experiences or life after death, so we knew our findings would be subjected to skepticism, flat-out disbelief and ridicule. But one case alone convinced me. A twelve-year-old girl told me that she had hidden her death experience from her mother. It had, she explained, been such a pleasant experience that she did not want to come back. "I don't want to tell my mommy that there is a nicer home than ours," she said.

Eventually she told her father all the details, including how she had been lovingly held by her brother. That shocked him. Until then, when he admitted as much, she had never known that she actually did have a brother. He had died a few months before she was born.

While we thought about what to do with our findings, our lives continued to move in separate directions. Both of us had been looking around for situations outside the stifling atmosphere of the hospital. The Reverend Gaines left first. In early 1970, he took over a church in Urbana. He also adopted the African name Mwalimu Imara. All the while I hoped that I would be the one who went sooner, but until I could leave I had to continue the seminars.

They were not something I could do as well without my one-of-a-kind partner. His old boss, Pastor N., took over. But there was such a lack of chemistry between us one student mistakenly thought Pastor N. was the doctor and I was the spiritual counselor. It was dismal.

I was getting ready to quit, and finally the Friday arrived when I decided that was going to be the last Death and Dying seminar of my career. I was always one for extremes. Afterward I approached Pastor N., preparing myself for how I was going to tell him that I was quitting. We stood by the elevator, reviewing the seminar that had just ended and discussing some new business. When he pushed the button to summon the elevator, I decided I had to seize the moment, resign before he got in and the doors shut. Then it was too late. The elevator doors opened.

I had just started to speak when a woman suddenly appeared between the elevator and Pastor N.'s back. My jaw dropped open. This woman hovered in the air, almost transparent, and she smiled at me as if we knew each other. "God, who is that?" I asked in a weird voice. Pastor N. had no idea what was going on. Judging by the way he was looking at me, Pastor N. thought I was losing my mind. "I think I know this woman," I said. "She's staring at me."

"What?" he asked, glancing around and seeing nothing. "What are you talking about?"

"She's waiting until you go into the elevator, and then she will come," I said.

The whole time Pastor N. had probably been planning his escape. He jumped into that elevator as if it were a safety net. The moment he was gone, this woman, this apparition, this vision, came straight toward me. "Dr. Ross, I had to come back," she said. "Do you mind if we walk to your office? I only need a few minutes."

Just a few dozen yards to my office. But it was the strangest, most exciting walk I had ever taken. Was I having a psychotic episode? I had been under some stress, but certainly not enough to be seeing ghosts. Especially ghosts who stopped outside my office, opened the door and let me enter first as if I was the visitor. But no sooner did she shut the door than I recognized her.

"Mrs. Schwartz!"

What was I saying? Ten months earlier Mrs. Schwartz had died. And been buried. Nevertheless, she was there in my office, standing beside me. She looked her usual pleasant but preoccupied self. Definitely not feeling that way myself, I sat down before I fainted. "Dr. Ross, I had to come back for two reasons," she said clearly. "Number one is to thank you and the Reverend Gaines for all you have done for me." I touched my pen, papers and coffee cup to make sure they were real. Yes, as real as the sound of her voice. "However, the second reason I came back is to tell you not to give up your work on death and dying . . . not yet."

Mrs. Schwartz moved to the side of my desk and offered me a radiant smile. That gave me a moment to think. Was this really happening? How did she know I was planning to quit? "Do you hear me? Your work has just begun," she said. "We will help you." Although it was hard for even me to believe it was happening, I could not prevent myself from saying, "Yes, I hear you." All of a sudden I sensed that Mrs. Schwartz already knew my thoughts and everything I was going to say. I decided to ask for proof that she was really there by giving her a pen and a sheet of paper and asking her to compose a brief note for the Reverend Gaines. She scribbled a quick thank-you. "Are you satisfied now?" she asked.

Truthfully, I did not know what I was. A moment later, Mrs. Schwartz vanished. I searched all over for her, found nothing, then ran back to my office and examined her note, touching the paper, analyzing the handwriting and so on. But then I stopped myself. Why doubt it? Why keep questioning?

As I have learned since then, if you are not ready for mystical experiences, you will never believe them. But if you are open, then you not only have them, and believe in them; people can hang you by your thumbnails and you will know that the experiences are absolutely real.

All of a sudden the last thing in the world I wanted to do was quit work. Although I still left the hospital a few months later, I went home that night energized and excited about the future. I knew Mrs. Schwartz had prevented me from making a terrible mistake. Her note went to Mwalimu. As far as I know, he still has it. For the longest time, he remained the only person whom I told about my encounter. Manny would have chided me like all the other doctors. But Mwalimu was different.

We soared to a different plane. Until then, we had been trying to define death, but now we looked beyond that, to an afterlife. Even though he had his new church, we struck a deal. Both of us agreed to continue interviewing patients and collecting data on life after death. I had work to do. After all, I had promised Mrs. Schwartz.

PART III

"THE BUFFALO"

CHAPTER TWENTY-SIX

Jeffy

In the middle of 1970 Manny suffered a mild heart attack. While he was in the hospital, I assumed that I would have no problem taking our children, Kenneth and Barbara, to visit him. After all, Manny worked there as a consultant and the hospital itself boasted of giving their staff seminars based on my book. There was reason to expect some real advances in the way patients and their families were treated. But the first time I took the kids to see their daddy, we were stopped outside the coronary unit by a guard who said, "No children are allowed."

Rejection? I could handle that, no problem. On the way into the hospital, I had noticed some construction in the parking lot. I led the kids back outside, turned on a flashlight and then guided them through a courtyard that led straight to a spot underneath Manny's window. From there we held up signs and waved. But at least the children saw that their father was okay.

Such extreme measures should have been unnecessary. Children went through the same stages of loss as adults. If not assisted, they got stuck and developed severe problems that could have easily been prevented. At Chicago Hospital, I watched a little boy ride up and down in the elevator. At first I thought he might be lost, but then I realized he was hiding out. Finally he noticed me staring and reacted by throwing several scraps of paper on the floor. When he was gone, I gathered up those scraps, pieced them together and saw he had written, "Thanks for killing my dad." Just a few visits could have helped him prepare for the loss.

But I was one to talk. A month before I finally quit the hospital, one of my dying patients asked why I never worked with dying children. "Damn if you aren't right," I exclaimed. Even though I devoted all my free time to being a mom to Kenneth and Barbara, who were growing into nice, smart kids, I avoided working with dying children. It was ironic, considering I had wanted to become a pediatrician.

The reason for my aversion was no secret once I thought about it. Every time I had contact with a terminally ill child, I saw either Kenneth or Barbara, and the thought of losing one of them was inconceivable to me. Yet I got over that hurdle by taking a job at La Rabida Children's Hospital. There I had to work with very sick, chronically ill and dying children. It was the best thing I had ever done. Soon I regretted not having worked with them from the start.

They were even better teachers than adults. Unlike older patients, the children had not accumulated layers of "unfinished business." They did not have a lifetime of botched relationships or a résumé of mistakes. Nor did they feel compelled to pretend that everything was okay. They knew instinctively how sick they were, or that they actually were dying, and they did not hide their feelings about it.

Tom, a chronically ill little boy, is a good example of the type of child I worked with there. He had never come to grips with always having to be in the hospital with kidney problems. Nobody had listened to him. As a result, he was filled with rage. He did not communicate. Nurses were frustrated by him. Rather than sit by his bed, I walked him out to a nearby lake. Standing on the shore, he hurled rocks into the water. Pretty soon he was ranting about his kidney and all the other problems that prevented him from having the life of a normal little boy.

But after twenty minutes, he was a different child. My only trick had been to give him the comfort to express his pent-up feelings.

I was also a good listener. I remember a twelve-year-old girl who was hospitalized with lupus. She was from a very religious family and her biggest dream was to spend Christmas at home with them. I understood the significance, and not just because Christmas was also special to me. But her doctor refused to let her leave the hospital, worrying that even a slight cold could end up being fatal. "What if we work hard to make sure she doesn't catch one?" I asked.

When that did not change his mind, the girl's music therapist and I wrapped her in a sleeping bag and smuggled her out through a window and to her home, where she sang carols all night. Though she returned to the hospital the next morning, I had never seen a happier child. Several weeks later, after she died, her strict physician admitted he was glad that her most important wish had been fulfilled.

On another occasion, I helped the staff deal with guilt over the sudden death of a teenage girl. Even though she was so ill that she was confined to strict bed rest, she was not too sick to develop a mad crush on one of the occupational therapists. She had wonderful spirit. When the staff threw a Halloween party on the ward, she attended, as a special treat, in a wheelchair. It was a wild affair, with loud music, and in a burst of spontaneity she got out of her wheelchair to dance with her favorite guy. Then suddenly, after a few steps, she dropped dead.

Needless to say, the party ended, and everyone suffered tremendous guilt. When I spoke with the staff, in a group session, I asked them what would have meant the most to this girl—living a few more months as an invalid or dancing with her true love in the midst of a great party? "If she had any regrets, it was that her dance wasn't longer," I said.

Isn't that true with life in general? But at least she got to dance.

Accepting the fact that children die is never easy, but I learned that dying children, much more than adults, tell you exactly what they need to be at peace. The biggest difficulty is being able to hear them. My all-time best example concerns Jeffy, a nine-year-old boy who had struggled with leukemia for most of his life. I have told his story countless times over the years, but it has proved so beneficial, and, like a dear friend, Jeffy is so much a part of my life, that I am going to repeat some of my recollections about him from my book *Death Is of Vital Importance:*

[Jeffy] was in and out of the hospital. He was a very sick boy when I saw him for the last time in the hospital. He had central nervous system involvement. He was like a drunk little man. His skin was

189

very pale, almost discolored. He was barely able to stand on his feet. He had lost his hair many, many times after chemotherapy. He could not even look at the injection needles anymore, and everything was too painful for him.

I was aware that this child had a few weeks, at the most, to live. That day it was a young, new physician who came on his rounds. As I walked in I heard him say to Jeffy's parents, "We are going to try another chemotherapy."

I asked the parents and the physician if they had asked Jeffy if he was willing to take another series of treatments. As the parents loved him unconditionally, they allowed me to ask Jeffy this question in their presence. Jeffy gave me a most beautiful answer in the way children speak. He very simply said, "I don't understand you grown-ups. Why do you have to make us children so sick to get us well?"

We talked about that. This was Jeffy's way of expressing the natural fifteen seconds of anger. This child had enough self-worth, inner authority and self-love to have the courage to say, "No, thank you," which was what Jeffy said to the chemotherapy. The parents were able to hear it, respect it and accept it.

Then I wanted to say goodbye to Jeffy. But Jeffy said, "No, I want to be sure that I am taken home today." If a child tells you, "Take me home today," there is a sense of great urgency, and we try not to postpone it. Therefore I asked the parents if they were willing to take him home. The parents had enough love and courage to do that. And again I wanted to say goodbye. But Jeffy, like all children who are still terribly honest and simple, said to me, "I want you to come home with me."

I looked at my watch, which in the symbolic, nonverbal language means, "You know, I don't have the time to go home with all my children." Without my saying anything in words, Jeffy understood instantly and said, "Don't worry, it will only take ten minutes."

I went home with him, knowing that in the next ten minutes Jeffy would finish his unfinished business. We drove home—the parents, Jeffy and I. We drove into the driveway, opened the garage. In the garage we got out of the car. Jeffy said very matter-of-factly to his father, "Take my bicycle down from the wall."

Jeffy had a brand-new bicycle that was hanging on two hooks

inside the garage. For a long time, the dream of his life had been to be able, once in his lifetime, to ride around the block on a bicycle. And so his father had bought him a beautiful bicycle. But because of his illness, he had never been able to ride it. It had been hanging on those hooks for three years. Now Jeffy asked his father to take it down. With tears in his eyes, he asked his father to put the training wheels on the bicycle. I do not know if you appreciate how much humility it takes for a nine-year-old boy to ask for training wheels, which are usually only for little children.

And the father, with tears in his eyes, put the training wheels on his son's bicycle. Jeffy was like a drunken man, barely able to stand on his feet. When his father finished putting on the training wheels, Jeffy took one look at me and said, "And you, Dr. Ross, you are here to hold my mom back." Jeffy knew that his mom had one problem, one piece of unfinished business. She was not yet able to learn the love that can say "no" to her own needs. Her biggest need was to lift up her very sick child onto the bicycle like a two-year-old, to hold on to him and to run with him around the block. This would have cheated him out of the greatest victory of his life.

Therefore I held his mom back, and her husband held me back. We held each other back and learned the hard way how painful and difficult it is sometimes to allow a vulnerable, terminally ill child the victory and the risk to fall and hurt and bleed. But then Jeffy drove off.

After an eternity, he came back. Jeffy was the proudest man you have ever seen. He was beaming from one ear to the other. He looked like somebody who had won an Olympic gold medal. He very proudly came off the bicycle and with great authority asked his father to take the training wheels off and to carry the bicycle into his bedroom. Then, very unsentimentally, very beautifully and very straightforwardly, Jeffy turned to me and said, "And you, Dr. Ross, you can go home now."

Two weeks later his mother called me up and said, "I have to tell you the end of the story."

After I left, Jeffy said, "When my brother comes home from school"—his brother Dougy was a first grader—"you send him upstairs. But no grown-ups, please." When Dougy came home he

191

was, as requested, sent up to his brother's room. A while later Dougy came back down but refused to tell his parents what he and his brother had talked about. He promised to keep it a secret until after his birthday in two weeks. In the meantime, Jeffy died the week before. Dougy had his birthday and then shared what had up till then been a secret.

In his bedroom, Jeffy had told his brother that he wanted the pleasure of personally giving him his most beloved bicycle. But he could not wait another two weeks until Dougy's birthday because by then he would be dead. Therefore he wanted to give it to him now.

But only under one condition: Dougy would never use those damn training wheels.

Back when I was first starting my work with dying patients, doctors accused me of exploiting people who they claimed were beyond hope. They were the ones who did not listen when I argued that dying patients could be helped, and even healed, right up until the end. It had taken almost ten years of hard work, but Jeffy's story, and the many thousands of others that occurred because of the work I did and inspired, was the sort they could not help but hear.

CHAPTER TWENTY-SEVEN

Life After Death

Until 1973, I helped dying children at La Rabida make the transition between life and death. At the same time, I assumed the responsibility of director of the Family Service Center, a mental health clinic. I thought the worst anybody could say about me was that I tried to do too much. But I underestimated. One day the clinic's chief administrator saw me treating one poor woman and later reprimanded me for counseling patients who could not afford to pay. That was like telling me not to breathe.

I was not about to stop that practice. If you hired me, you also got what I stood for. For the next couple of days, we debated the issue. While I argued that doctors had a responsibility to treat needy patients regardless of their ability to pay, he said that he had a business to run. Eventually he tried to compromise, offering to let me take care of charity cases on my lunch hour. But to make sure he could keep track of how I managed my time, he ordered me to punch a time clock.

No thanks. I quit and, at age forty-six, I suddenly had the time to pursue new, exciting projects like my first Life, Death and Transition workshop, which was an intensive weeklong series of group lectures, interviews with dying patients, Q&A sessions and one-on-one exercises geared toward helping people overcome the tears and anger in their lives—what I described as their old unfinished business. This could be the death of a parent that was never mourned, sexual abuse never admitted or some other trauma.

But once expressed in a safe environment, the healing process began and people were able to live the kind of open, honest lives that enabled a good death.

Soon I had offers to give these workshops around the world. About 1,000 letters came to the house each week. The phone seemed to ring just as frequently. My family felt the growing pressures that my popularity put on us, but they were supportive. My research into life after death took on an unstoppable momentum. Throughout the early 1970s, Mwalimu and I interviewed about 20,000 people who fit that profile, ranging in ages from two to ninety-nine years old and including cultures as diverse as Eskimos, Native Americans, Protestants and Muslims. In all cases the experiences were so similiar that the accounts had to be true.

Up till then I had absolutely no belief in an afterlife, but the data convinced me that these were not coincidences or hallucinations. One woman, who had been pronounced dead after a car crash, said she came back after seeing her husband. Later, doctors told her that he had died in a separate car accident across town. In another case, a man in his thirties described how he had committed suicide after losing his wife and children in a car wreck. Once dead, though, he saw his family, who were all okay, and he returned.

Not only were we told that the death experience was free of pain; people reported that they did not want to come back. After being met by loved ones, or guides, they traveled to a place that was so loving and comforting that they did not want to return. They had to be talked into it. "It's not time," was something practically everyone heard. I remember watching a five-year-old boy draw a picture in an effort to explain to his mother how pleasant his death experience had been. First he drew a brightly colored castle and said, "This is where God lives." Then he added a brilliant star. "When I saw the star, it said, 'Welcome home.'"

These remarkable findings led to an even more remarkable scientific conclusion that death did not exist—not in its traditional definition. I felt any new definition had to go beyond the death of the physical body. It had to consider the proof we had that man also had a soul and spirit, a higher reason for life, a

194

poetry, something more than mere existence and survival, something that continued on.

Dying patients went through the five stages, but then after "we have done all the work we were sent to Earth to do, we are allowed to shed our body, which imprisons our soul like a cocoon encloses the future butterfly," and . . . well, then a person had the greatest experience of his life. It did not matter if the cause of death was a car accident or cancer (though someone who died in a plane crash or a similarly sudden, unexpected incident might not know right away he is dead), at death there was no pain, fear, anxiety or sorrow. Only the warmth and calm of a transformation into a butterfly.

According to the interviews I compiled, death occurs in several distinct phases.

PHASE ONE: In the first phase, people floated out of their bodies. No matter if someone flat-lined in an operating room or died in a car wreck or committed suicide, everybody reported being totally aware of the scene he or she had left. They floated out of their bodies like butterflies leaving their cocoon. They assumed an ethereal shape. They knew what was happening, heard discussions other people were having, counted the number of doctors working on them or saw the effort being made to free them from mangled vehicles. One man reported the license plate number of the hit-and-run car that smashed into him. Others recounted what their relatives had said at their bedside at the time of death.

In this first phase, they also experienced a wholeness. For instance, if somebody had been blind, his sight returned. If they had been paralyzed, they now moved effortlessly and joyously. One woman told how she had enjoyed dancing above her hospital room so much that she had been severely depressed when she had to come back. Indeed, the only complaint from the people I spoke to was that they did not stay dead.

PHASE TWO: At this point, people had left their bodies behind and reported being in a state of life after death that can only be defined as spirit and energy. They were comforted to discover that no human being ever dies alone. No matter where or how they had died, they were able to go anywhere with the speed of thought. Some reported thinking of how upset their family members were going to be by their death and then, zoom, they were with them, even if they were halfway around the world. Others who had been in ambulances remembered visiting with friends at work.

I found this phase to be the most comforting to people who had to grieve over the death of a loved one, especially a sudden, tragic death. It is one thing for someone to wither away over a long period of time from cancer. Everyone—patient and family—has time to prepare for the eventuality of death. A plane crash is not so easy. Those who die are as confused as their families and in this phase they get time to figure out what happened. For instance, I am positive those who died aboard TWA flight 800 were with their families at the memorial service on the beach.

Everyone I interviewed remembered this phase for also being when they met their guardian angels, guides, or—as children often referred to them—playmates. They described their angels as being like guides, comforting them with love and introducing them to the presence of previously deceased parents, grandparents, relatives or friends. It was remembered as a time of cheerful reunion, sharing, catching up and hugs.

PHASE THREE: Guided by their guardian angel, my subjects then proceeded into the third phase, by entering what has commonly been described as a tunnel, or a transitional gate, though people recounted a variety of different images—a bridge, a mountain pass, a pretty stream—basically whatever was most comfortable to them. They created it with psychic energy, and at the end they saw a bright light.

As their guides took them closer, they felt the light radiating intense warmth, energy, spirit and love. Love most of all. Unconditional love. People reported that its force was overwhelming. They felt excitement, peace, tranquillity and the anticipation of finally going home. The light, they said, was the ultimate source of the universe's energy. Some called it God. Others said it was Christ or Buddha. But everyone agreed on one thing—they were enveloped by overwhelming love. It was the purest of all love, unconditional love. After listening to thousands and thousands of people describe this same journey I understood why none of them wanted to return to their physical bodies.

But those who did come back reported that it had the same profound effect on their lives. It had been like a religious experience. Some had been given great knowledge. Some had come back with prophetic warnings. Others had new insight. But everyone experienced that same epiphany of thought—that seeing the light had taught them that there is only one explanation for the meaning of life, and that is love.

PHASE FOUR: In this phase, people reported being in the presence of the Highest Source. Some called it God. Others reported simply knowing they were surrounded by every bit of knowledge there was, past, present and future. It was nonjudgmental and loving. Those who arrived here no longer need their ethereal shape. They become spiritual energy, the form human beings assume between lives and when they finish their destiny. They experienced a oneness, a completeness of existence.

In this state, people went through a life review, a process in which they confronted the totality of their lives. They went over every action, word and thought of their lives. They were made to understand the reasons for every decision, thought and action they had in life. They saw how their actions affected other people, including strangers. They saw what their lives could have been like, the potential they had. They were shown that everybody's life is intertwined, that every thought and action has a kind of ripple effect on every other living thing on the planet.

I interpreted this as being heaven or hell. Maybe both.

The greatest gift God gave man was free choice. But that requires responsibility—the responsibility to make the right, the best and the most thoughtful, respectful choices, choices that benefit the world, choices that improve mankind. In this phase, people reported being asked, "What service have you rendered?" It was the hardest question to answer. It demanded that people confront whether or not they had made the highest choices in life. They found out whether or not they learned the lessons they were supposed to learn, the ultimate being unconditional love.

The basic conclusion I drew, and one that has remained

unchanged, is that human beings, whether rich or poor, American or Russian, have similar needs, wants and concerns. In fact, I have never met a person whose greatest need was anything other than love.

Real unconditional love.

You can find it in a marriage or in a simple act of kindness toward someone who needs help. But there is no mistaking love. You feel it in your heart. It is the common fiber of life, the flame that heats our soul, that energizes our spirit and supplies passion to our lives. It is our connection to God and to each other.

Every person goes through struggles in life. Some are great and some do not seem so important. But they are the lessons we have to learn. We do that through choice. In order to have a good life, and thus a good death, I tell people to make their choices with the goal of unconditional love, by asking, "What service am I rendering?"

Choice is the freedom God has given us; the freedom to grow and love.

Life is a responsibility. I had to choose whether or not to counsel a dying woman who could not afford to pay. I made my choice based on what I felt in my heart was the right thing to do, even though it cost me my job. That was fine with me. There would be other choices. Life is full of them.

Ultimately, each person chooses whether he comes out of the tumbler crushed or polished.

CHAPTER TWENTY-EIGHT

Proof

For six months in 1974, I stayed up late at night pounding out my third book, *Death: The Final Stage of Growth*. From the title alone, you would have thought that I had all the answers about death. But on the day I finished, September 12, my mother died in the Swiss nursing home where she had spent the past four years and I found myself asking God why He made this woman, who, for eighty-one years, gave only love, shelter and affection, a vegetable and kept her in that state for so long. Even at her funeral, I cursed Him for His unkindness.

Then, as unbelievable as it sounds, I changed my mind and was actually thanking Him for his generosity. It sounds insane, right? It did to me too—until it dawned on me that my mother's final lesson had been to learn how to receive affection and care, something she had never been good at. From then on, I praised God for teaching her in just four years. I mean, it could have been a lot longer.

Though life unfolds chronologically, lessons come when you need them. Just the previous Easter I had gone to Hawaii to lead a workshop. People looked upon me as the expert on life. And what happened? I ended up learning an immensely important lesson about myself. It was a great workshop, but a miserable time because the man who had organized it was a real cheapskate. He had booked us into a horrible place, complained that we ate too much and even charged for the paper and crayons we used.

On my way back home, I stopped in California. Friends

picked me up at the airport and asked how the workshop had been. I was so distraught I could not answer. So attempting to be funny, they said, "Tell us about your Easter bunnies." For some reason, I heard that and started to cry uncontrollably. All the anger and frustration that I had repressed the previous week came spewing out. That kind of behavior just was not typical of me.

Later that night, once safely tucked away in my room, I analyzed what had caused that outburst. The mention of Easter bunnies had triggered the memory I had of the time my father told me to take Blackie to the butcher.

Suddenly all the pain, anger and unfairness that I had repressed for nearly forty years came flooding out. I cried the tears that I should have cried then. I also realized that I had an allergy to cheap men. Every time I met one, I became tense, subconsciously reliving the death of my favorite bunny. Finally, this penny-pincher in Hawaii pushed me to the point of explosion.

Not surprisingly, once those feelings were externalized, I felt much better.

It is impossible to live life at the highest level unless you get rid of your negativity, your unfinished business . . . your black bunnies.

If there was another black bunny inside me, it was my need—as a "two-pound nothing"—to constantly prove myself worthy of being alive. At forty-nine, I was unable to slow down. Manny was also busy building his reputaton. There was not much time for a healthy relationship. The perfect antidote, I thought, would be to buy a farm, some out-of-the-way place where I could recharge my batteries, relax with Manny and give the children experiences with nature similar to those I had as a child. I envisioned lots of acreage, trees, flowers and animals. If Manny did not share my enthusiasm, at least he recognized that the car trips we took looking at farms were chances to be together.

On our last outing of the summer of 1975, we found the perfect site in Virginia. It had fields out of a picture book, including sacred Indian mounds. I loved it. Manny seemed equally keen, judging by the way he snapped pictures of the place with an expensive camera he had borrowed from a friend. We talked about it in the car as Manny took me to a hotel in Afton, where

I was going to lead a workshop starting the next day. After dropping me off, Manny and the kids were driving back to Chicago.

Yet on the way into town, we passed a strange-looking little house. A woman who had been standing on her porch ran out toward our car waving her arms frantically. Thinking she needed help, Manny stopped the car. It turned out that the woman, a complete stranger, knew where I was staying that night and was waiting for me to pass by her house on the way to the hotel. She asked me to follow her into the house. "I have to show you something very important," she said.

As odd as that sounds, it was not unusual—not for me. By that time, I was used to people going to great lengths to talk to me or saying they desperately needed to ask me a question. Since I always tried to be accommodating, I told this woman she had two minutes. Once she agreed, I followed her into the house. She took me into a small, cozy living room and pointed to a photograph on a table. "There," she said. "Look." At first glance, the picture was merely a pretty flower, but then I looked closer and saw that the flower was being used as a perch by a creature with a small body, face and wings.

I turned toward the woman. She nodded. "It's a fairy, isn't it?" I said, feeling my heart start to beat faster.

"What do you think?" she replied.

Sometimes it pays not to think with your head as much as with your instinct, and this was one of those times. At this point in my life, I was open to anything and everything. Most days I felt as if a curtain was being lifted to give me access to a world no one had ever seen before. This was proof. It was one of those great turning points. Normally I would have asked for a cup of coffee and talked this woman's head off. However, my family was out in the car. I did not have time for questons. I accepted the photo as it was.

"Do you want an answer that's honest or one that's polite?" I said.

"Never mind," she said. "That gives me your answer."

Before I even moved toward the door, she handed me a Polaroid camera, motioned toward a back door that led to a well-manicured backyard garden and told me to photograph any of the plants or flowers. To appease her and get myself out of there, I snapped one shot and pulled out the film. A few seconds later, another flower fairy came into focus. Part of me was amazed. Part of me wondered what the trick was. And still another part of me quickly thanked her and rejoined Manny and the children, although when they asked what the woman had wanted I made up a story. Sadly, there were more and more things I couldn't tell my family.

Before leaving me at the hotel, Manny handed me his borrowed camera, thinking it was safer for me to hand-carry this expensive item on the plane rather than risk its being stolen out of the motel where they planned to stop at night. He lectured me on the importance of taking good care of high-priced equipment, a spiel I'd heard so many times before I didn't bother to listen again. "I promise not to touch it," I said while putting it over my shoulder and later chuckling at the paradox of my promise not to touch it while at the same time draping it over me.

Once I was alone, I immediately thought of the fairies. I first heard of fairies in the stories I read as a child and I also talked to my plants and flowers, but neither made me believe that fairies existed. On the other hand, I couldn't stop thinking about that odd woman who photographed the fairies. That was powerful, provocative evidence. So was the fact that I'd been able to do the same thing with her Polaroid camera. If it was a trick, it was a damn good one. But I didn't think it was fake.

Ever since Mrs. Schwartz's visit, I knew better than to discount something because I could not explain it. I believed that everyone was watched over by a guide or guardian angel. Whether on the battlefields of Poland or in the barracks of Maidanek or the hallways of a hospital, I had often felt guided by something more powerful than me.

And now fairies?

If you are ready for mystical experiences, you have them. If you are open, you will have your own spiritual encounters.

No one could have been more open than I was when I got back to my hotel room. Taking the camera that belonged to Manny's friend—the forbidden fruit, since I had promised not to touch it—I drove to a grassy field on the edge of the woods, found a clearing in front of a slight rise and sat down. The scene reminded me of my secret childhood hideout behind our house in Meilen. There were three shots left on the roll of film in the camera.

Three shots: On the first try, I aimed at the hill in front of me, which had woods in the background. Before taking the second photo, I called out, as in a dare, "If I do have a guide and you can hear me, make yourself visible in the next picture." Then I snapped the picture. The final shot was wasted.

Back at the hotel, I repacked the camera and promptly forgot about my experiment. About a month later, my memory was jarred. I was rushing to catch a flight from New York to Chicago, carrying an enormous bag of treats for my Brooklyn-born husband—a dozen Kuhn's kosher hot dogs, several pounds of kosher salami and New York-style cheesecake. By touchdown, the entire plane smelled like a delicatessen. I dashed home to surprise Manny, who didn't expect me till later that night. As I prepared dinner, he called looking for one of the kids. Instead of sounding happy when I answered, he snapped, "Well, you did it again."

"Did what again?" I asked. I had no idea what he meant. "The camera," Manny snapped. I had no clue what camera he meant. Annoyed, he explained that it was the expensive camera that he'd borrowed and entrusted to me in Virginia. "You must've used it," he said. "I got the pictures developed and there's one shot at the end that is double-exposed. The damn thing has got to be ruined." Suddenly I remembered my experiment. Ignoring Manny's criticism, I begged him to hurry home. As soon as he walked through the door, I asked for the pictures like an impatient child.

If I hadn't seen the pictures with my own eyes, I never would have believed what was on them. The first was of the meadow and the woods. The second was the same exact scene but super-imposed on the foreground was a tall, muscular, stoic-looking Indian with his arms folded across his chest. As I shot the photo, he looked straight at the camera. His expression was very serious. No kidding around.

I was ecstatic, turning somersaults inside. Those pictures were items that I would treasure and keep my entire life. They were hard evidence. Unfortunately, they were destroyed, along with all my other pictures, diaries, journals and books, when my house was burned down in 1994. But then I could only stare at them and marvel. "So it is true," I said softly.

Manny, set to scold me again, asked what I had muttered. "Oh, nothing," I said. It was too bad that I did not feel comfortable sharing all the excitement with my husband, but he would not have tolerated such a waste of his time. He had problems accepting my studies about life after death. And fairies? Well, the days when we supported each other through medical school and the long hours of our difficult residencies were in the past. Now that Manny was fifty, with a history of heart trouble, he was interested in settling down and owning lots of things. In many ways I was just beginning.

That would be a problem.

CHAPTER TWENTY-NINE

Channeling the Other Side

I had gotten assistance. Now I needed help. I had found proof that life continued after death. There were also pictures of fairies and guides. Pieces of a whole new, uncharted world had been shown to me. I felt like an explorer nearing the end of a long voyage. Land was in sight. Still, I could not get there by myself. I really wished there was someone to go to, I told people in my ever-widening circle of connections, someone who knew more.

Sure, the tofu-eating mediators contacted me with all sorts of offers about talking to the dead and traveling to higher planes of consciousness. But they were not my type. Then in early 1976 I was contacted by a couple in San Diego, Jay and Martha B., who promised to introduce me to spiritual entities. "You'll be able to talk to them," the B.s promised. "You can talk to them and they'll answer."

That got my attention. We spoke a number of times on the phone, then I booked a lecture in San Diego that spring and visited them.

At the airport, the three of us embraced like old friends. Jay B., a former aircraft worker, and his wife, Martha, were about my age and looked like any ordinary middle-class couple. He was balding; she was plump. They took me to their house in Escondido, where they had a good thing going. Since founding their self-named Church of Divinity the previous year, they had developed a core following of about a hundred people. The big attraction was B.'s ability to channel spirits. A channeler goes into a deep state of mind or trance to summon the knowledge of a higher spirit or deceased wise person. His sessions were held in a little building, or the "dark room," behind their house. "We call it the 'phenomenon of materialization,'" he said excitedly. "I can't begin to share all the lessons we've been given so far."

Who could blame me for my excitement? On my first day there, I joined twenty-five people of all ages and types in the dark room, a squat windowless building. Everyone sat on folding chairs. B. placed me in the front row, a spot of honor. Then the lights were switched off and the group began singing, a soft, rhythmic hum that built to a loud group chant, which gave B. the energy needed to channel the entities.

Despite my anticipation, I was still reserving the right to be skeptical, but, as the chanting reached a new, almost euphoric level, B. disappeared behind a screen. Suddenly an enormously tall figure appeared to the right of me. He was a shadowy sort of figure. But compared with Mrs. Schwartz, he had more density and a more imposing presence. He was seven feet tall and spoke in a deep voice. "By the end of the evening, you will be amazed but more confused," he said.

I already was. Sitting on the edge of my seat, I fell under his captivating spell. It was incredible, yet I wondered if I was experiencing the greatest moment of my life. He sang, greeted the group and then zeroed in on me, until he towered right over me. Everything he did and said was deliberate and meaningful. He called me Isabel, which would make more sense a few minutes later, and then he told me to be patient, because my soul mate was trying to make it.

Although I wanted to ask what soul mate, I could not speak. Then he disappeared, and after a long, dark moment, another, altogether different figure materialized. He introduced himself as Salem. Like the first spirit, he bore no similarity to the Indian I had photographed before. Salem was tall and slender, dressed in a long, flowing robe and a turban. Quite an individual. As he moved in front of me, I said to myself, "If this guy touches me, I'm going to drop dead." At the instant I had that thought, Salem disappeared. Then the first figure came back and explained that my nervousness had made Salem go away.

Five minutes passed, enough time for me to calm down. Then

Salem, my so-called soul mate, reappeared right in front of me. Though my thoughts had scared him off, he decided to test me by putting his toes on the front tip of my Birkenstock sandals. When that failed to frighten me, he leaned even closer. I could tell he was being careful not to frighten me, and he wasn't. As soon as I wished that he would move a little faster, get to the point, he officially introduced himself, greeted me as his "beloved sister, Isabel," and then gently got me up from my chair and led me into a pitch-dark back room where we were alone.

Salem acted strange and mystical while also being calming and familiar. Warning me that he was about to take me on a special journey, Salem explained that in another lifetime, the time of Jesus, I had been a wise and respected teacher named Isabel. Together, we traveled back to a pleasant afternoon when I had sat on a hillside, listening to Jesus preach to a group of people.

Although I visualized the whole scene, I could barely understand Jesus and asked, "Why the hell can't he talk normal?" But as soon as I said that, it dawned on me that my dying patients, like Jesus, often communicated in a symbolic language, like parables. If you are tuned in, you can hear it. If not, you miss out.

Nothing got by me that evening. After an hour, I was on overload, almost glad the session ended so I could let the whole experience settle. There was a lot to digest, more than I ever expected. At my lecture, which I delivered the next day, I threw out my prepared talk and shared what had happened the night before. Instead of getting criticized for being nuts, the reaction I expected, the audience gave me a standing ovation.

Later that night, my last one before going back home to Chicago, B. took me into the dark room again—by myself. There was a part of me that wanted to see it again, to make sure everything was kosher. This time it took a little longer for B. to channel, but Salem eventually appeared. As we said hello to each other, I sat there wishing my mother and father had been able to see how far their littlest daughter had gone in life. Suddenly Salem started to sing the words to "Always . . . I'll be loving you . . ." No one other than Manny knew that song was a Kübler family favorite.

"He's quite aware," Salem said, referring to my father. "He knows."

A day later, back in Chicago, I told Manny and the kids every-thing. They sat with open mouths. Manny listened without passing judgment; Kenneth seemed interested; Barbara, then thirteen, was the most outwardly skeptical, maybe even a little frightened. Whatever reaction they had was understandable. This was way-out stuff for them and I did not hold back anything. But I hoped Manny, and perhaps Kenneth and Barbara, would keep an open mind and maybe one day even meet Salem in person.

Over the next few months I returned frequently to Escondido and met spirits other than Salem. One particular guide named Mario was an absolute genius who spoke eloquently about what-ever subject I raised, whether it was geology, history, physics or crystals. But my bond was with Salem. "The honeymoon's over," he said one night. Evidently that meant heavier, more philo-sophical discussions, because from then on Salem and I spoke mostly about ideas like natural and unnatural emotions, child rearing and healthy ways of externalizing grief, anger and hate. Later I was able to incorporate these theories in my workshops.

But incorporating them into my home life was another matter. It should have been a time of celebration. There I was, on the cut-ting edge of research that would change and improve an untold number of lives. But the deeper I went, the harder it was for my family to accept it. The scientist in Manny had trouble accepting anything to do with life after death. In fact, there were many arguments over whether or not, as he believed, the B.s were taking advantage of me. Kenneth was old enough to approve of his mother, as he said, "doing her own thing," while Barbara resented the time I spent working.

I guess I was too involved to notice the strain my work caused in the family until it was too late. I hoped someday to reconcile these worlds. Such a dream seemed possible if I could ever find a farm, an idea that still interested me.

But then that dream was shattered. One morning, after I'd left to catch a plane to Minneapolis, Salem called the house. How many times had I desired to have a conversation with Salem from home? Now he called, and instead of me, Manny answered. It was the worst thing in the world. He didn't understand channeling, no matter how clearly I explained it. His logical mind would not let him. It was the stuff of great arguments. To him, Salem sounded like a strange man disguising his voice. "How can you believe that garbage?" he said. "B. is taking advantage of you."

Things seemed to have gone back to normal when we put in an indoor swimming pool. I took many relaxing midnight dips after returning from lectures. And there was nothing as indulgent as swimming when the snow piled up outside the glass windows. On a few occasions the whole family even enjoyed splashing and laughing together in the water. However, that happy sound was short-lived. On Father's Day in 1976, after the children and I took Manny out for a fancy Italian dinner, we stood in the parking lot and he explained why dinner had been so tense. He wanted a divorce. "I'm leaving," he said. "I rented an apartment in Chicago."

At first I thought Manny was playing a joke. Then he drove off without so much as hugging the children. Somehow I did not see us as a divorced family, one of those statistics. I tried assuring Kenneth and Barbara that their father would return. I told myself that Manny would miss my cooking, need his laundry done or want to entertain his hospital friends in the garden now that it was in full bloom. But then one night, as I opened the back door for Barbara and a friend, a man jumped out of the bushes and handed me a copy of the divorce papers that Manny had filed in court the day before.

Once when I was not home Manny came back. I found the mess around the pool from a party he had hosted. That made how he felt about me obvious. But I was not going to fight. Barbara needed a stable home life, somebody who could be there with her every night, and that was not me. I told Manny he could have the house, packed some essentials, just clothing, books and bedding, in boxes and shipped them to Escondido. I had no idea where else to go until I knew what to do with my life.

Needing support, I flew to San Diego for a day and conferred with Salem. He gave me the sympathy I desperately needed as well as the type of guidance I hoped for. "What would you think about having your own healing center on top of a mountain near here?" he asked. Naturally I said yes. "So it shall be," he said.

There was one more trip back to my Frank Lloyd Wright home in Flossmoor, where I said my goodbyes, worked one last time in my kitchen and tearfully tucked Barbara into bed. Then

I moved into my new address, a trailer home, in Escondido. It was tough starting over at fifty years old, even for someone like me who had the answers to life's big questions. My trailer was too small to hold my books or even fit a comfortable chair. Few friends called to help. I felt lonely, isolated and deserted.

Gradually the good weather proved to be my savior by drawing me into the healthy outdoors. I planted a vegetable garden and took long, contemplative walks through eucalyptus groves. The B.s' friendship alleviated my loneliness and inspired me to look forward. After a month or two, I started to bounce back. I bought an adorable little house with a sun porch overlooking a lovely meadow, plenty of room for my books and a hillside which I covered with wildflowers.

Once the urge to work returned, I made plans to start my own healing center. As it moved beyond the talking phase, I tried to make sense of the weird turn of events that caused my marriage to end and me to move across the country, where I was on the verge of the biggest undertaking of my life. It was impossible. I just reminded myself that there are no accidents. Now that I felt better, I could help others again.

Thanks to Salem's guidance, I found the perfect site on which to build the center—forty acres above Lake Wohlfert, a gorgeous view included. As I surveyed the property, a monarch butterfly landed on my arm, a sign telling me to look no further. "This is the place where we need to build," I said. It was not so easy, something I discovered when I applied for a loan. Since Manny had always handled all our money, I had no credit rating. Even though I had a good income from my lectures, no one would give me a loan. The insanity almost drove me to sympathize with the feminist movement.

But my single-mindedness and lack of business sense won out. In exchange for the Flossmoor house, all the furniture, and some child support, Manny agreed to pay for the healing center property and lease it back to me. Soon, once a month, I was leading weeklong workshops that helped medical and nursing students, terminally ill people and their families deal with life, death and transition in a healthier, more open manner.

The workshops, initially limited to forty people at a time, had a long waiting list. Wanting to heal people in all dimensions of life, I asked the B.s, my closest confidants and supporters, to lend their talents to the project. Although they had no financial stake in the healing center, I treated them like partners. Martha supervised psychodrama classes, developing exercises that helped people break through repressed episodes of anger and fear. She really showed talent. But her husband's channeling sessions continued to be the most impressive and powerful events.

He was a powerful channeler with a natural charisma. The core group of church followers remained staunch devotees. But with more and more outsiders attending sessions, B. occasionally had to defend himself against people who believed his channeling was a hoax. He met those challenges by issuing a stern warning: if anyone turned on the lights while he was channeling, they risked harming the spirits—and quite possibly him too. Yet once, as B. channeled an entity named Willie, a woman turned on the lights. The sight was unforgettable—B. stark naked.

B. remained in his trance, while the rest of the room went into a panic over Willie's health, but he was later able to explain that was his method of making the spirit materialize through him. Nothing to worry about.

I was skeptical of a guide named Pedro. I do not know why, but some sixth sense, which I had learned to trust, told me he might be a fake. I investigated the next time the spirit appeared by asking him questions only a genius could answer, questions that I knew were beyond B.'s knowledge. Not only did Pedro handle them without hesitation; he tried to climb atop a wooden horse that was used by the psychodrama workshop, joked that it was too high for him, disappeared and then returned a moment later a half foot taller. Then he looked at me and said, "See, I know you're skeptical."

After that I had no problem with Pedro's credibility. He was at his best outside the workshops, when it was just the old group. In those sessions he became more intimate with each person, offering advice on issues in their personal lives. "It had been hard for you, Isabel, but you had no choice." As helpful as he could be, I noticed a negativity creep into his repertoire. He warned that the future held changes that would split the group and challenge B.'s credibility. "It's up to each one of you to make your own choice," he explained. Later I realized he was addressing rumors of strange, sometimes sexually abusive goings-on in the dark room, but I was not aware of those stories then. I traveled so much that I was often out of the gossip loop.

As for the future, I did not worry about it, since it would come whether I liked it or not, but Pedro often seemed to be preparing me more than anyone else for a change. "Free choice is the highest gift man received when he was born into planet Earth," he said. "Every moment you make choices, in your speaking, doing and thinking, all of them are terribly important. Each choice affects every life form on the planet." Even if I did not understand why something was being said at these sessions, I learned to accept it. Guides only provided knowledge. It was up to me, like everyone else, to decide how to use it. Thus far, it had done well by me. "Thank you, Isabel," Pedro said, getting down on one knee in front of me. "Thank you for accepting your destiny."

I wondered what that would be.

CHAPTER THIRTY

Death Does Not Exist

K nowing that I was so busy that my lectures were booked a year or two in advance, a friend once asked how I managed my life, how I made my decisions. My answer surprised her. I said, "I do what feels right, not what's expected." That explained why I still talked with my ex-husband. "You divorced me, I didn't divorce you," I would tell him. That was also the reason I decided to make an unscheduled stop in Santa Barbara while heading to a lecture in Seattle. I suddenly felt like visiting an old friend.

You had to expect things like that from a woman who told people to live each day as if it could be their last. My friend was delighted when I phoned her. Indeed, I was expecting a nice afternoon visit over tea. But when my friend's sister met me at the airport she said there was a change in plans.

"They don't want me to say anything about it," she said apologetically.

The mystery was cleared up soon enough. My friend and her husband, a well-known architect, lived in a pretty Spanish-style house. As soon as I walked through the door they embraced me and expressed relief that I had actually made it. Was there a possibility I might not? Before I had time to ask if anything was wrong, they led me into the living room and pushed me into a chair. My friend's husband sat opposite me and rocked himself back and forth into a trance. I gave my friend a questioning look. "He's a channeler," she said.

Hearing that, I knew confusion would straighten itself out,

and so I shifted my attention back to her husband. His eyes were closed, his expression quite serious and as the spirit took over his body he looked as if he had aged a hundred years. "It worked to bring you here," he said, his voice now strange, urgent and old. "It's important that you no longer procrastinate. Your work with death and dying is completed. It's now time for you to begin your second assignment."

Listening to patients or channelers was never a problem for me, but understanding what they said sometimes took awhile. "What do you mean, my second assignment?" I asked.

"It's time for you to tell the world that death does not exist," he said.

Although guides are there solely to help you complete your destiny and fulfill the promises you made to God, I protested. I needed more explanation. I needed to know why they had picked me. After all, I was known throughout the world as the Death and Dying Lady. How could I possibly turn around and tell the world death did not exist? "Why me?" I asked. "Why don't you pick a minister or someone like that?"

The spirit grew impatient. I was quickly reminded that I chose my work in this lifetime on Earth. "I am merely telling you it is time," he said. Then he launched into a huge list of reasons why it was me and no one else they had in mind for this special assignment, ticking them off one by one: "It had to be a person from medicine and science, not from theology and religion, since they had not done their job and had ample opportunity in the last two thousand years. It had to be a woman and not a man. And someone who was not afraid. And someone who reached a lot of people and could give them the feeling she talked to them personally . . .

"That's it. It is time," he finally concluded. "You have a lot to digest."

No question about that. After a cup of tea, my friend, her husband and I, totally drained physically and emotionally, retired to our bedrooms. Once by myself, I realized that I had been summoned for this specific reason. Nothing happened by chance. And hadn't Pedro already thanked me for accepting my destiny? As I lay in bed, I wondered what Salem would have to say about this assignment.

214

No sooner did I think that than I felt someone else in my bed. My eyes opened.

"Salem!" I exclaimed.

It was dark, but I saw that he had materialized from the waist up. "The energy was so high in this house that I was able to put it together for just a couple of minutes," he explained. I marveled at having summoned him without B.'s help, something that made me feel less dependent on B. Obviously, B. no longer had a lock on these special moments. "Congratulations on your second assignment, Isabel," Salem added in his deep familiar voice. "I wish you well."

Before leaving, Salem massaged my spine and sent me into a deep sleep. Back home, I put together all of the knowledge and experiences I had gained over the years concerning life after death. Not long after, I gave my new lecture, titled "Death and Life After Death," for the first time. It was as nerve-rattling as the first time I took Professor Margolin's place at the podium. But the reaction was overwhelmingly positive, which proved I was on the right path. During one lecture in the Deep South, I was taking questions, after interviewing a dying man, when a woman, probably in her early thirties, caught my eye. "Yours will be the last question," I said. She hurried to the microphone. "Please tell me, what do you think a child experiences at the moment of death?"

This was a perfect opportunity to summarize the lecture. I described how children, similar to adults, leave their physical body just like a butterfly emerges from a cocoon, then go through the different stages of life after death that I had described earlier. Then I mentioned that Mary often helps when children are involved.

Like a bolt of lightning, the woman raced to the stage, where she told how her little boy, Peter, suffering from a bad cold, had an allergic reaction to a shot given him by his pediatrician and died in the examining room. As she and the pediatrician waited for "what seemed like an eternity" for her husband to arrive from work, Peter miraculously opened his large brown eyes and said, "Mommy, I was dead and with Jesus and Mary. There was so much love. I didn't want to come back. But Mary told me that it was not my time."

Although Peter ignored her, Mary took his hand and declared, "You have to get back. You have to save your mommy from the fire."

At that instant, Peter returned to his body and opened his eyes.

The mother, who was sharing this story for the first time since it happened thirteen years earlier, admitted that she lived in a state of misery and depression from knowing that she was doomed to "the fire," or as she interpreted it, doomed to hell. She had no idea why. After all, she was a good mother, wife and Christian. "It doesn't seem fair," she cried. "It has ruined my entire life."

It was not fair, but I knew I could help lift her depression quickly by explaining that Mary, like other spiritual beings, often spoke symbolically. "That's the problem with religions," I said. "Things are written so they can be interpreted or, in many cases, misinterpreted." I told her that I was going to prove my point by asking her some questions, which I wanted her to answer without pausing to think: "What would it have been like if Mary had not sent Peter back to you?"

She grabbed her hair and looked horrified. "Oh my God, I would've gone through hell and fire," she said.

"Do you mean you would have walked through fire?" I asked.

"No, that's an expression," she explained.

"Now do you see?" I asked. "Do you see what Mary meant when she told Peter he had to save you from the fire?"

Not only did she see, but over the next few months, as my lectures and workshops gained in popularity, I saw that people were more than ready to accept life after death. Why not? The message was positive. Countless people shared similar experiences of leaving their body and traveling toward a bright light. They were so relieved to finally have these stories confirmed. It was life-affirming.

But the stress of all the changes of the past six months—my divorce, buying a new house, starting a healing center and virtually circling the globe giving lectures—were taking their toll. Without a break, it was too much wear and tear. Finally, after a speaking tour through Australia, I took some time for myself. I desperately needed to. With two couples, I booked an isolated mountain cabin. It did

216

not have any phones or mail delivery, and poisonous snakes kept people off the grounds. It was heavenly.

After a week, the daily chores of rustic life, like chopping firewood for the stove and fireplace, had begun to make me feel like a decent, rested person again, and I still looked forward to another week, after my friends left. Then I would be all by myself—perfect. But the night before the two couples were to depart, they voted to stay with me. I went to bed depressed.

In the darkness, emotionally depleted and depressed, I had the urge to cry out for help. So many people looked to me to solve their troubles, but who did I have for affection and support? Although I had never called on my spirits outside of Escondido, they had promised to come if I ever needed them.

"Pedro, I need you," I said softly.

Despite the distance between Australia and San Diego, in less than an instant my favorite spook Pedro appeared in my cabin bedroom. Although he already knew my thoughts, I still asked if I could cry on his broad shoulder. "No, you cannot do that," he said firmly. In the same breath, he added, "But I can do something else for you." Slowly he extended his arm, then put my head in the palm of his outstretched hand and said, "When I leave you will understand." While he and I were alone, I had the sensation of being carried away in the palm of his hand. It was the most beautiful and satisfying feeling of peace and love I had ever experienced. All my concerns disappeared.

Without any parting remarks, Pedro quietly walked away. I had no idea how late it was, if the night had just begun or dawn was near. It didn't matter. In the darkness, my eyes fell upon a little wooden statue that was on my bookshelf. It was of a child comfortably nestled in the palm of a hand. All of a sudden I was enveloped by the same feelings of protectedness, care, peace and love as I had been when Pedro touched his hand to my head, and I fell asleep on a huge pillow on the floor.

When my friends woke me the next morning, they wondered why I had not gone to bed. Still, they commented on how rested I finally looked. I was unable to tell them anything about what had happened during the night, since I was still overwhelmed by it. But Pedro had been right. I understood. Millions of people in the world had mates, lovers, partners and so on. But how many others had the thrill and comfort of being carried in the palm of His hand?

No, I would no longer complain or feel sorry for myself for not having a shoulder to cry on. In my heart, I knew that I was never alone. I had received what I needed. Frequently, as I had on that night, I longed for a companion, for some love, for a hug or a shoulder to lean on—something I never found.

But I received other gifts, which few people ever experienced, and if I could have traded them, I would have refused. That I knew.

Judging from what had happened recently, I had no doubt anymore that much of life is finding out what you already know. That is particularly true with spiritual experiences and powers. Take the lesson I learned from Adele Tinning, an elderly woman in San Diego who had talked with Jesus daily for seventy years. They spoke through her heavy oak kitchen table, which lifted and lurched beneath the spot where she placed her hands, spelling out messages in a kind of Morse code.

Once, while my sisters were visiting, I took them to Adele's. As we sat around her table, which was so heavy that the three of us could not have budged it even if we had wanted to, Adele shut her eyes and giggled softly. Then the table started to sway under her fingertips. "Your mother is here," she said, opening her sparkling brown eyes. "She says to wish you happy birthday." My sisters were shocked. None of us had mentioned that it was also our birthday.

A few months later I was able to perform the feat myself. One night, as I was preparing a veal dinner, my two houseguests—nuns from Texas, one of whom was blind—took their car to the pharmacy on an errand, normally a ten-minute round trip. When they were not back after a half hour, I began to worry. I sat down at the kitchen table and wondered what to do. "Should I call the police?" I asked out loud. "Could they have been in an accident?"

Suddenly, the table moved slightly, bumped and slipped, and then I heard someone say in a loud voice, "No." I nearly hit the ceiling. "Am I talking with Jesus?" I asked. Again the table moved and I heard the same voice say, "Yes." The mind-boggling experience was just beginning when the back door opened and

218

the two nuns appeared. Seeing what was happening, they grinned. "Oh, you can do the table too?" Sister V. exclaimed, pulling out a chair for herself. "Let's do it together." It was the best thing I had ever cooked up in the kitchen.

Which is not to say that I felt satisfied. Soon I was leading a workshop in Santa Barbara. On the final night of what had been an intense five days, I did not get back to my cabin until 5 A.M. As I got into bed, barely able to keep my eyes open, a nurse dashed in and asked to watch the sunrise with me. "Sunrise?" I screamed. "Be my guest. Watch it here, but I'm going to sleep."

A few seconds later, I was in a deep sleep. But instead of "falling" asleep, I felt as if I was rising up out of my body, higher and higher, but without any control or fear. Once aloft, I perceived several beings take hold and carry me off to someplace where they fixed me up. It was like having several car mechanics work on me. Each had their own specialty—brakes, transmission and so on. In no time, they had replaced all the damaged parts with new ones and set me back in bed.

In the morning, after just a few hours' sleep, I woke up feeling blissfully serene. The nurse was still in my room, so I told her what had happened. "You obviously had an out-of-body experience," she said. I gave her a puzzled look. After all, I did not meditate or eat tofu. Nor was I a Californian. Nor did I have a guru or a Baba. My point? That I had absolutely no idea what she was talking about when she said "out-of-body experience." But if they were anything like that, I was ready for another flight anytime.

CHAPTER THIRTY-ONE

My Cosmic Consciousness

After my out-of-body experience, I made a trip to the library and found one book on the subject. This author's name was Robert Monroe, the famous researcher, and soon I arranged to take another trip, this time to Monroe's Virginia farm, where he has built his own research laboratory. For years, the only kind of mind experiments anyone heard of were all related to drugs, which I was against. So imagine my excitement when I saw Monroe's setup—a modern lab full of electronic equipment and monitors, the kind of stuff that gave me an immediate sense of credibility.

I was there to have another out-of-body experience. To do that, I entered a soundproof booth, lay down on a water bed and slipped a blindfold over my eyes, shutting out all light. Then an assistant fitted a set of earphones over my head. To induce the experience, Monroe had devised a method of stimulating the brain through iatrogenic means—or artificial sound pulses. These pulses caused the brain to go into a meditative state and then even beyond—the destination I sought.

My first try, though, was somewhat disappointing. The lab supervisor turned on the machine. I heard the steady sound of a beeping in my ears. The rhythmic pulses started out slowly and then quickly sped up, till they were one rapid indistinguishable high-pitched sound, which took me very quickly into a sleeplike state of mind. It was apparently too quickly, according to the lab supervisor, who brought me back down after a few moments and asked if I was all right.

"Why'd you stop?" I asked, perturbed. "I felt like I was just starting."

Later that day, though a bowel obstruction I'd been suffering from for a few weeks was causing me discomfort, I climbed onto the water bed for a second chance. Because scientists are a cautious bunch by nature, I was careful to exert more influence this time. I stipulated that they throw the switches to full speed. "No one has ever traveled that fast," the lab supervisor warned.

"Well, that's the way I want it," I said.

Indeed, this second time was the experience I wanted. It is hard to describe, but the beeping instantly cleared my mind of all thoughts and took me inward, like the disappearing mass of a black hole. Then I heard an incredible WHOOSH, similiar to the sound of a strong wind blowing. Suddenly I felt as if I was swept up by a tornado. At that point I was taken out of my body and I just blasted away.

To where? Where did I go? That is the question that everyone asks. Although my body was motionless, my brain took me to another dimension of existence, like another universe. The physical part of being was no longer relevant. Like the spirit that leaves the body after death, similar to the butterfly leaving its cocoon, my awareness was defined by psychic energy, not my physical body. I was simply *out there*.

Afterward, the scientists in the room asked me to describe the experience. While I would have liked to provide details, which I knew were extraordinary, I was not helpful. Other than telling them that my bowel obstruction had suddenly cleared up, along with a slipped disk in my neck, and that I felt okay, not dazed or tired or anything, I said, "I don't know where I was."

That afternoon, feeling strange and wondering if I had gone too far, I returned to the guesthouse on Monroe's ranch where I was staying, an isolated cabin called the Owl House. As soon as I entered, I sensed a strange energy, which convinced me that I was not alone. Since the house was secluded and without a phone, I thought about returning to the main house for the night or going to a motel. But, believing there are no coincidences, I realized that my hosts had put me out by myself for a reason. So I stayed.

Despite efforts to stay awake, I got into bed and fell fast

asleep—and that is when the nightmares began. They were like going through one thousand deaths. They tortured me physically. I could barely breathe, and I bent over in agony and pain so overwhelming that I did not even have the strength to scream or call for help, even though no one would have heard me if I had. During the hours this lasted, I noticed that each time a death was completed another one began, without any break in between to breathe, recuperate, scream or prepare for the new one. One thousand times.

The point was clear. I was reliving the deaths of all the patients I had attended up till that time, reexperiencing their anguish, grief, fear, suffering, sadness, loss, blood, tears. . . . If somebody had died of cancer, then I felt their agonizing pain. If someone had a stroke, then I suffered the effects too.

I received three reprieves. The first time I asked for a man's shoulder to lean on. (I had always liked falling asleep on Manny's shoulder.) But the moment I expressed my need, I heard a deep, manly voice respond, "You shall not be given!" The denial, given in a firm, determined and emotionless tone, did not allow time to ask another question. I would have liked to ask, "How come?" After all, my shoulder had been leaned on by so many dying patients. But there was no time, energy or space for it.

Instead the pain and suffering, gripping me like nonstop labor pains, returned to such a degree that I simply hoped to pass out. I had no such luck, though. There is no telling how much time passed before I was granted a second reprieve. "May I have a hand to hold?" I asked. I purposely did not specify a man or a woman. Who had time to be choosy? I just wanted a hand to hold. But the same firm, unemotional voice again turned me down, saying, "You shall not be given!"

I had no idea there would be a third respite, but when it came, trying to be sneaky, I took a deep breath and got set to ask to be shown a fingertip. My thinking? While you cannot hold a fingertip, it at least proves the presence of another human being. But before I expressed this last request, I said to myself, "Hell, no! If I cannot get a single hand to hold, I don't want a fingertip either. I would rather do it without help and on my own."

Angry and resentful, mustering every bit of defiance in my will, I said to myself, "If *they* were so cheap they wouldn't even give me a hand to hold, then I would be better off alone. At least I would have my self-esteem and self-worth on my own terms."

That was the lesson. I had to experience all the horror of one thousand deaths in order to reaffirm the joy that came afterward.

Suddenly, getting through the ordeal, like life itself, became a matter of FAITH.

Faith in God—that He would never send anything to anybody that they could not handle.

Faith in myself—that I could handle anything that God would send, that no matter how painful and agonizing, I would be able to see it through.

I had an awesome feeling that someone was waiting for me to say something, say the word "yes." Then I knew that was all that was being asked of me—to say yes to it.

My thoughts raced.

What did I say yes to? More agony? More pain? More suffering without human assistance?

Whatever it was, nothing could be worse than what I had already endured, and I was still here, wasn't I? Another hundred deaths? Another thousand?

It mattered little. Sooner or later there would be an end to it. Besides, by then the pain was so intense that I could no longer feel it. I was beyond pain.

"Yes," I shouted. "YES!"

The room got still, and all the pain, agony and breathlessness ceased in an instant. Almost completely awake, I noticed it was dark outside. I took a deep breath, the first substantial one in no telling how long, and glanced once more out the window into the dark night. I took another breath, relaxed while lying on my back and then began noticing some peculiar things. First a section of my abdomen, one that was clearly delineated, began to vibrate at an ever-increasing speed, but this motion was unrelated to the muscles, which caused me to say, "That cannot be."

But it was, and the more I observed my own body lying there, the more amazed I became. Whatever part of my body I looked at began to vibrate with the same fantastic speed. The vibrations broke everything down to their most basic structure, so that when

224

I stared at anything, my eyes feasted on the billions of dancing molecules.

At this point, I realized that I had left my physical body and become energy. Then, in front of me, I saw many incredibly beautiful lotus blossoms. These blossoms opened very slowly and became brighter, more colorful and more exquisite, and as time passed they turned into one breathtaking and enormous lotus blossom. From behind the flower, I noticed a light—brighter than bright and totally ethereal, the same light that all my patients talked about having seen.

I knew that I had to make it through this giant flower and eventually merge with the light. It had a magnetic pull, which drew me closer and gave me the sense that this wonderful light would be the end of a long and difficult journey. Not in any hurry, thanks to my curiosity, I indulged in the peace, beauty and serenity of the vibrating world. Surprisingly, I was still aware of being in the Owl House, far away from any contact with other humans, and whatever my eyes landed on vibrated—the walls, ceiling, windows . . . the trees outside.

My vision, which extended for miles and miles, caused me to see everything, from a blade of grass to a wooden door, in its natural molecular structure, its vibrations. I observed, with great awe and respect, that everything had a life, a divinity. All the while, I continued to move slowly through the lotus flower, toward the light. Finally, I was merged with it, one with the warmth and love. A million everlasting orgasms cannot describe the sensation of the love, warmth and sense of welcome that I experienced. Then I heard two voices.

The first was my own, saying, "I am acceptable to Him."

The second, which came from somewhere else and was a mystery to me, said, "Shanti Nilaya."

Before falling asleep that night, I knew that I would awake before sunrise, put on a pair of Birkenstocks and a robe which I had carried in my suitcase for weeks but never worn. This handwoven robe, which I had purchased at Fisherman's Wharf in San Francisco, felt like one that I had worn previously, perhaps in another lifetime, so when I bought it I had the sense of reclaiming it.

The next morning everything happened as I had envisioned. While walking along the path toward Monroe's house, I continued to see every leaf, butterfly and stone vibrating in its molecular structure. It was the greatest feeling of ecstasy a human being can experience. I was so filled with awe for everything around me, and in love with all of life, that, like Jesus, who was able to walk above the water, I walked above the stones and pebbles on the path, even going so far in my blissful state as to tell them, "I cannot step on you. I cannot hurt you."

Gradually, over several days, this state of grace diminished. It was very difficult to return to mundane household chores and driving a car, which all seemed so trivial afterward. Soon I would be told the meaning of Shanti Nilaya and also that the whole experience was supposed to give me Cosmic Consciousness, an awareness of the life in every living thing. To that end, it was successful. But what else? Was there another painful separation to go through with practically no help from human beings until I found my own answers and a new beginning?

Months later, when I traveled to Sonoma County, in California, for a workshop, I started to get some answers. But I nearly made a decision that could have cost me that understanding. The physician who had agreed to take care of the physical needs of the workshop's terminally ill patients in exchange for my lecturing to a transpersonal psychology conference he had organized in Berkeley, canceled at the last minute. Naturally, after leading the grueling workshop by myself, I assumed my obligation to him was annulled.

But on Friday, as the last of my workshop participants drove off, a friend called to tell me that several hundred people had signed up for my lecture. On the drive to Berkeley, he reiterated the level of enthusiasm awaiting me, trying to pep me up. But exhausted from my own workshop, I shared little of the excitement and, in all honesty, had absolutely no idea what I was going to say to the sophisticated and highly evolved group of people attending the conference. Yet once in the auditorium, I knew that I had to speak about what I had experienced back at Monroe's ranch. Someone there would explain it to me.

Starting out by saying that I would share my own spiritual

evolution, I warned that I would need some help from them in figuring out everything, since much of it was beyond my intellectual understanding. In a joking manner, I emphasized that I was not "one of them"—I did not meditate, nor was I a Californian or a vegetarian. "I smoke, drink coffee and tea, and in short I am a regular person," I said, getting a big laugh.

"I have never had a guru or visited a Baba," I continued. "Yet I have had almost every mystical experience anybody could wish for." My point? If I could have these experiences, then anybody could have them without going to the Himalayas to meditate for years.

By this time, as I discussed my first out-of-body experience, the room was dead silent. After two hours, I wrapped up with a thorough account of having died one thousand deaths and then been reborn at the Monroe ranch. There was a long, standing ovation. Then a monk, clad in an orange robe, approached the stage with great reverence and offered to clarify some things I said. First, he said that while I might think that I could not meditate, there were many forms of meditation. "When you sit with dying patients and children and focus on them for hours, you are in one of the highest forms of meditation," he said.

There was more applause, which verified his opinion, but the monk paid no mind, as he was focused on delivering one more message. "Shanti Nilaya," he said clearly, pronouncing each lovely syllable slowly. "It is Sanskrit, and it means 'the final home of peace.' It's where we go at the end of our earthly journey when we return to God."

"Yes," I said to myself, echoing the words I had heard in the dark room months before. "Shanti Nilaya."

CHAPTER THIRTY-TWO

The Final Home

I was back home, standing on my balcony. The B.s had come over for tea. A warm breeze gently massaged our senses. Feeling the intoxication of fate, I faced my neighbors and in a somewhat ceremonious tone of voice announced that the healing center would be named Shanti Nilaya. "It means 'the final home of peace,'" I explained.

That seemed to strike the right note. For the next year and a half, well into 1978, Shanti Nilaya thrived. Concerned with "the promotion of psychological, physical and spiritual healing of children and adults through the practice of unconditional love," the five-day, live-in Life, Death and Transition workshops quadrupled their enrollment. There was an increasing population hungry for personal growth. My newsletter was circulated around the world, and I kept pace with a personal travel schedule that took me from Alaska to Austria.

Even as Shanti Nilaya grew, its purpose remained narrow—personal growth. In workshops people got rid of their unfinished business, all the rage and anger they experienced in life, and learned how to live so they were ready to die at any age. In other words, they became whole. Typical workshops included dying patients, people with emotional troubles and ordinary adults ranging from age twenty to a hundred and four; before long I added workshops for teenagers and children. The sooner a person became whole, the better chance he or she had to grow up to be physically, emotionally and spiritually healthy.

Wouldn't that bode well for the future?

Those who came into contact with me, whether at Shanti Nilaya or on the road, all heard more or less the same thing. "Death is nothing to fear. In fact, it can be the most incredible experience of your life. It just depends on how you live your life now. And the only thing that matters right now is love."

My most helpful work resulted from contact with a nine-year-old boy I met while lecturing in the South. During these long talks, as my energy went through ups and downs, I would recharge myself by engaging with people in the audience. I spotted Dougy's parents in the front row. Although I had never seen them before, my intuition told me to ask this pleasant-looking young couple where their child was. "I don't know why I feel the need to say this," I said, "but why didn't you bring him here?"

Surprised that I would ask such a question, they explained that he was receiving his chemotherapy treatment at the hospital. After the next break, though, the father returned with Dougy, who bore the signs of cancer—thin, pale and bald—but otherwise looked like an all-American boy. Dougy colored with crayons and paper while I continued speaking. Afterward, he gave me the picture as a present. No one ever gave me a better one.

Like most dying children, Dougy was wise beyond his years. Because of his physical suffering, he had developed a keen understanding of his spiritual, intuitive abilities. That is true of all dying children and it's why I urge parents to share their anger, pain and grief honestly and openly with them. They know everything. And one look at Dougy's picture reconfirmed that for me. "Shall we tell them?" I asked, motioning to his parents.

"Yeah, I think they can take it," he said.

Dougy's parents had recently been told that their son had only three more months to live. Their biggest problem was accepting that news. But from the drawing, I was able to contradict that diagnosis. As far as I could tell from what he had drawn, Dougy had much longer to live, maybe three years. His mother, overcome with joy, hugged me. Yet I could take no credit. "I am only a translator reading this drawing," I said. "It's your son who knows those things."

What I loved about working with children was their honesty.

They cut through all the phony baloney. Dougy was a perfect example of that. One day I received letter from him. It said:

Dear Dr. Ross,
    I have only one more question left: What is life and what is death and why do little children have to die?
Love, Dougy

Taking some felt-tipped markers, I created a colorful booklet that drew on all my years of work with dying patients. In simple language, I described life as a gamble, similar to the scattering of seeds in a windstorm, covered by earth and warmed by the sun, whose rays were God's love shining down on us. Everyone had a lesson to learn, a purpose to his or her life, and I wanted to tell Dougy, who would die three years later and was trying to figure out why, that he was no exception.

Some flowers bloom only for a few days—everybody admires and loves them as a sign of spring and hope. Then they die—but they have done what they needed to do . . .

There have been many thousands of people who have been helped by that letter. But it is Dougy who deserves all the credit.

I wish that I had had as much insight into the problems brewing on the home front. In early spring 1978, while I was on the road, some of our friends who had regularly attended B.'s sessions with our teacher-guides, discovered a book called *The Magnificent Potential*, which had been written twenty years earlier by a local man named Lerner Hinshaw. The book contained everything that B. and many, though not all, of the guides he channeled had taught over the past two years. As soon as I heard, I was, like everyone else, stunned and betrayed.

When questioned, B., denying any wrongdoing, argued that the guides prohibited him from divulging the source of his knowledge. A confrontation was to no avail. Each one of us was left to act as judge and jury. Over half the group left, disillusioned and unable to trust any longer. As for me, I did not know what to do and found myself haunted by Pedro's warning to me

231

months earlier. "It's up to each one of you to make your own choice," he had said. "Free choice is the highest gift man received when he was born into planet Earth."

Like me, those who remained did not want to give up the incredibly meaningful teachings of the guides, but once our suspicions were aroused, we noticed certain irregularities in the sessions. New people disappeared into the back room for long periods of time. We heard giggling and curious noises. I wondered what sort of instruction was being given. Then one day a friend of mine came to my house, crying, distraught and looking for refuge from B. After calming down, she reported that B. had told her it was time to deal with her sexuality. That caused her to fall apart and flee.

There was no choice except to confront B. and his wife, which we did the next day at my house. As on previous occasions, he showed no guilt or remorse. He obviously believed that he had done the right thing. His wife, though disturbed, was used to such behavior by him. Indeed, it turned out, upon further investigation, that he had a history of creepy behavior, and from then on we prevented anyone from being alone in a room with him without supervision.

But trouble continued. The San Diego branch of the state Department of Consumer Affairs received complaints, and then, in December, the District Attorney's office began investigating allegations of sexual misconduct. Despite numerous interviews, the DA's inquiry failed to produce any charges. As one investigator told me: "Everything took place in the dark. You have no proof."

That was a big dilemma, since we had been told repeatedly that a materialized entity would die if someone turned on a light in its presence. None of us wanted to take that chance. But I was seriously conflicted. If fake, how could those entities have the knowledge to answer all my questions, which were beyond B.'s limited education. Hadn't we also seen with our own eyes how an entity materialized in front of us? Hadn't Pedro made himself six inches taller in order to get on a wooden horse?

Assisted by a few trustworthy friends, I began my own investigation. But B. was very shrewd. Once, seconds before I was about to switch on a flashlight, he excused himself and declared the session finished. Another time, we handcuffed the channeler's arms behind his back to prevent him from moving and fooling around with the participants. Still, entities appeared and disappeared, and when the session finished, the channeler was still in handcuffs, only they were on his feet. All of our efforts ended like that.

Despite the dark cloud overhead, our regular evening sessions with B. continued in the dark room. Unfortunately, there was a noticeable decline in his once-powerful gifts as a healer, which only added to the tense atmosphere. I had many questions. Our group, previously close-knit, caring and sharing, was becoming suspicious and paranoid. Should I walk away? Or should I stay? I had to find the truth.

In the meantime, B. ordained me a minister of peace in his church. Although every little thing B. did was now tinged with distrust, the evening was still an emotional, unforgettable event. All the entities appeared at the celebration, including K., the highest of all the entities. We always knew when he arrived—a strange silence preceded his entrance, and once he stood in front of us, in a long Egyptian-style robe, no one was able to move. I could not move a finger, not even an eyelid.

Ordinarily K. spoke few words, but this time he described my life as an example of working for love and peace. "Since your secret wish has always been to be a true minister of peace, tonight your wish will be fulfilled," he said. He let Pedro perform the actual ritual while Salem played the flute.

A few months later, while I was speaking to two friends outside, K. appeared suddenly, standing seven feet above the ground against a tall building. There was no mistaking his beautiful Egyptian robe or his loud and clear voice. "Isabel, in the river of tears, always count your blessings," he said. Then, just before disappearing, he added, "Make time your friend."

That left me shocked. More tears? Did I not have enough pain from losing my family? My children? My home? And then my trust in B.?

"Make time your friend."

What did that imply? That in time things would get better? Did I just have to wait patiently?

You could tell from my schedule that patience was not one of my virtues. Trying to keep an eye on B. at all times, I started taking him and his wife to my workshops. Not a thing happened. But one day on our way home from Santa Barbara, as B.'s wife and I waited by the car, he did not show up for over an hour. Then he was unapologetic. However, knowing I was exhausted from the workshop, B. put his jacket on the backseat and told me to sleep while he drove back to San Diego.

Halfway to Los Angeles, I fell into a deep sleep. I opened my eyes as we pulled into my driveway and then went right back to sleep on top of my bed.

About 3 A.M. I woke up with the feeling that I was sleeping on a big balloon rather than a pillow. I turned my head from side to side several times, but the strange feeling did not go away. Although woozy and confused, I groped my way to the bathroom, turned on the light and looked in the mirror. I nearly had a heart attack. My face looked completely disfigured. One side was as swollen as a big balloon, my eye pushed shut. The other eye was barely open, just enough to see. I looked grotesque. "What the hell happened?" I asked out loud.

I had a vague recollection of lying on the jacket in the car and feeling something bite me on the cheek. Actually, I had felt myself being bitten three times. But I had been too drowsy and sleepy to react. Now, on examining myself more closely, I saw three small but distinct bite marks on my cheek, and it looked like it was going from bad to worse. My face was continuing to swell even as I stood there. Since I lived too far from a hospital, and was in no condition to drive, and B., whom I did not trust, was my nearest neighbor, I faced a serious problem.

"You were bitten by a poisonous spider," I told myself calmly. "You don't have much time."

My thoughts raced. There was no time to call my family, who were spread across the country. Time was running out. I thought back to the hundreds of times when I thought that my life might come to an end. In times of great stress and sorrow, I had even pondered, if only for a second, suicide. In those moments, I would have loved to die a thousand times. But I could never do that to my family. The guilt and remorse would have been too much. No, I could never do that.

Nor did I ever lose a patient to suicide. Many had wanted to take their own lives, but I would ask them what it was about their

234

condition that made life unbearable. If it was pain, I increased the medication. If it was family problems, I tried to resolve them. If they were depressed, I tried to help them out of it.

The goal is to help people live until they die a natural death. I would never ever help a patient take his own life. I do not believe in assisted suicide. If a mentally competent patient refuses to take his medication or undergo her dialysis, there comes a point when we have to accept a person's right to do that. Some patients complete their unfinished business, put their affairs in order, reach a stage of peace and acceptance and rather than prolong the dying process take time into their own hands. But I would never assist them.

I have learned not to be judgmental. Ordinarily, if a patient has accepted death and dying, he is then able to wait for what comes naturally. It is then a very lovely and transcendental experience.

By committing suicide, a person may be cheating himself out of the lesson he is supposed to learn. Then, instead of graduating to the next level, he will have to return and learn that previous lesson from the beginning. For instance, if a girl takes her own life because she cannot live after breaking up with her boyfriend, she will have to come back and learn to deal with loss. In fact, she may have a life full of losses, until she learns to accept it.

For me, as my face continued to swell, just the thought that I actually had a choice kept me alive. What a strange thought that the choice of suicide actually kept me alive. There was no question, though, that is what happened. If I did nothing to combat my rapidly deteriorating condition, I would be dead in a few minutes. But I had a choice, the free choice God grants everyone, and I alone, at that instant, had to decide if I was going to live or die.

I walked into my living room, where a picture of Jesus hung on the wall. Standing before it, I made a solemn vow to live. The instant I said that, the room filled with an incredibly bright light. As I had done before when faced with that same bright light, I moved toward it. Once enveloped by the warmth, I knew that, no matter how miraculous it seemed, I would live. A week later, the bites were examined by a respected physician, who said, "They look like black widow bites. But if that was the case, you would not be alive." As far as I was concerned, he would never believe the treatment that had saved me, so I did not bother discussing it. "You're lucky," he said.

Lucky, yes. But I also knew that my real problems, rather than ending, had just begun.

CHAPTER THIRTY-THREE

AIDS

There is no problem that is not actually a gift. I had trouble believing that when I got word that Manny, apparently hard-pressed for money, sold the Flossmoor house without, as we had previously agreed, giving me the option to buy it, and then, in another painful and sneaky move, also sold the Escondido property that was home to Shanti Nilaya. A registered letter notified me that I had to empty the houses and hand the keys to the new owners. I was devastated beyond words.

Should I have felt any different? After losing my home, then having my dream yanked out right from under me, I cried myself to sleep many nights. It made no difference, did it, those words my spooks had advised: "In the river of tears, count your blessings. Make time your friend."

But then, a week later, San Diego was pounded by a torrential rainstorm that lasted for seven days. The downpour resulted in major flooding, mud slides and property damage, including my former mountaintop healing center. The roof of the main house collapsed, the swimming pool cracked and filled with mud and the steep access road was completely washed away. If we had still been there, not only would we have been stranded but the repairs would have cost a fortune. Strange as it seemed, my eviction had been a blessing.

I shared the good feelings with my daughter when she visited me over Easter. Barbara was a very intuitive girl who had never trusted B. or his wife. I always assumed that she blamed them for my move to California. Now, however, she was in college, a few years behind her brother at the University of Wisconsin, and we had a great relationship again.

Thank God for that. After settling into my house, which allowed her to take in the huge sun porch, the hot tub, the birds and the millions of flowers in bloom, we drove to apple orchards in the mountains, a lovely excursion that turned ugly on the way back when the brakes on my car gave out as I drove down the steep road. That we survived was nothing less than miraculous. We said the same thing a few days later. After driving a widowed friend of mine to her place in Long Beach, Barbara and I raced back to finish preparing our Easter feast and found my house engulfed by flames.

As huge flames tore through the roof, we sprang into action. I grabbed the garden hose while Barbara ran to the neighbors to call the fire department. She tried three different homes, but nobody answered. Finally, against her better judgment, she rang the bell at the B.s'. They opened the door and promised to call the fire department. But that was all they did. Neither of those supposed friends came by to offer help, which we definitely could have used, since Barbara and I, with our garden hoses, had put the fire out by the time the first truck arrived.

Once the firemen broke through a wall, we entered the house. It was a nightmare. The furniture was destroyed. All of the light fixtures, telephones and other plastic equipment had melted down. My wall hangings, Indian rugs, pictures and dishes were all black. The smell was unbearable. We were told not to stay inside there for any length of time, since the fumes were bad for our lungs. The odd thing was the turkey that I intended to serve for Easter dinner smelled delicious.

Uncertain what to do next, I sat on the car and smoked a cigarette. One of the really nice firemen came over and asked if he could recommend a counselor who specialized in helping people who lose everything in fires. "No, thanks," I said. "I am used to loss and I'm a specialist myself."

The next day the firemen returned to check on us, which I really appreciated. Still, neither B. nor his wife had come by. "Are they really your friends?" Barbara asked.

Someone did not like me. Or so it seemed, after both an arson investigator and a private detective concluded that the fire had started simultaneously in the kitchen stove and the woodpile outside the house. "There's at least a suspicion of arson," the investigator said. What was I to do? Spring cleaning came early. After Easter, the insurance company brought a big truck and moved the burned stuff away, including my grandmother's silver collection, which I had been saving for Barbara. Now it was just a big melted lump.

Some of my Shanti Nilaya friends helped me clean, wash and scrub everything that was still usable. The only thing not touched or even blackened by the fire was an old sacred Indian ceremonial pipe. Pretty soon, with money I received from the insurance company, I had an army of construction workers rebuilding the house. It was not the same house, though, and when it was done I would put it up for sale.

My faith was really being put to the test. I had lost my mountaintop healing center and my trust in B. The series of freakish incidents threatening my life—the spider bites, the brake failure and the fire—was too close for comfort. I believed my life was in danger. Was it worth it? After all, at the age of fifty-five, how much was I expected to keep giving before giving up? I felt I had to get away from B. and his evil energy. The thing to do was to buy that farm I had dreamed of for years, slow down and take care of Elisabeth for a change. Perhaps it was the right idea. But the timing was not quite right. Because in the midst of my own crisis of faith, I was pressed into service again.

It was called AIDS, and it changed the rest of my life.

For a few months I had heard rumors of a gay cancer. No one knew much about it except that once healthy, active and vibrant men were dying at an alarmingly fast rate, and they were all homosexual. As a result, no one in the general public was very alarmed.

Then I got a phone call from a man asking if I would accept an AIDS patient in my next workshop. Since I never turned any terminally ill patient down, I signed him up immediately. But a day and a half after meeting Bob, whose gaunt face and spindly limbs were covered with large, unsightly purple blotches—a deadly skin malignancy known as Kaposi's sarcoma—I caught myself praying to get away from him. My brain was screaming for answers: What does he have? Is it catching? If you help him, will you end up like him? Never in my life had I been more ashamed.

Then I listened to my heart, which encouraged me to see Bob as a suffering human being—a beautiful, honest, caring and loving man. From then on, I regarded it as a privilege to serve him, as I would any other human being. I treated him the way I would have liked to be treated if our positions had been reversed.

But my initial reaction scared me. If I, Elisabeth Kübler-Ross, who had worked with every kind of dying patient and literally written the book, had first been repulsed by this young man's condition, then I could not even imagine the struggle society would have in dealing with this pandemic called AIDS.

The only acceptable human reaction was compassion. Bob, twenty-seven years old, had no idea what was killing him. Like other young homosexual men with the disease, he knew he was dying. His fragile, deteriorating health kept him housebound. His family had deserted him long ago. His friends quit visiting. He was understandably depressed. One day in the workshop, he tearfully recalled how he had telephoned his own mother and apologized for being gay, as if he had any control over that.

Bob was my test. He was the first of thousands of AIDS patients whom I helped find peaceful closure to a tragic conclusion of life, but he actually gave much more in return. On the workshop's last day, the participants, including a rigid fundamentalist minister, serenaded Bob with a loving song and carried him around the room in a group embrace. Through his courage, we, in that workshop, received a greater understanding of honesty and compassion, which we carried out into the world.

We would need it. Because the people getting AIDS were overwhelmingly gay, the population's general attitude in the beginning was that they deserved to die. It was, in my opinion, a catastrophic denial of our own humanity. How could true Christians turn their back on AIDS sufferers? How could people in general not care? I thought back to how Jesus took care of leprosy patients and prostitutes. I recalled my own struggle to win rights for the terminally ill. Gradually we heard of heterosexual men, women and babies contracting the disease. In AIDS, all of us, whether we liked it or not, had to confront an epidemic that demanded our compassion, understanding and love.

At a time when our planet was threatened by nuclear waste, toxic dumping and war that could be greater than any in history, AIDS challenged us collectively as human beings, worldwide. If we couldn't find the humanity in our hearts to treat AIDS, then we were doomed. Later on I would write, "AIDS poses its own threat to mankind, but unlike war, it is a battle from within . . . Are we going to choose hate and discrimination, or will we have the courage to choose love and service?"

*   *   *

Talking to early AIDS patients, I became suspicious that they suffered from a man-made epidemic. In earlier interviews with AIDS patients, many of them mentioned receiving an injection that purportedly cured hepatitis. I never had time to investigate, but if that was true it only meant we had to fight that much harder against evil.

Soon I led my first workshop exclusively for AIDS patients. It took place in San Francisco, and, as I would many times in the future, I listened to one young man after another tell the same heartbreaking story of a life of deception, rejection, isolation, discrimination, loneliness and all the negative behavior of humanity. I didn't have enough tears in me to do all the crying that needed to be done.

On the other hand, AIDS patients were incredible teachers. None epitomized the potential for enlightenment and growth more than one particular Southern young man who participated in that original AIDS-only workshop. After being in and out of hospitals for a year, he looked like an emaciated Nazi concentration camp prisoner. From his condition, it was hard to call him a survivor.

Before dying, he felt compelled to make peace with his parents, whom he hadn't seen for years. He waited till his strength returned, then in a borrowed suit that hung on his bony frame like clothes on a scarecrow, he flew home. He was so worried that his physical appearance might disgust them, he considered turning around. But his parents spotted him. Rising from the porch where they nervously waited, his mother ran out, ignored the purple lesions dotting his face and embraced him without hesitation. His father followed. And they reunited, tearfully and lovingly, before it was too late.

241

"You see," this young man said on the last day of the workshop, "I had to have this dreadful disease in order to really know what unconditional love is all about."

All of us did. From then on, my Life, Death and Transition workshops opened up to AIDS patients across the country, and then throughout the world. To ensure that nobody was ever turned away for lack of money, since medication and hospitalization ate up so many life savings, I began knitting scarves, which were auctioned off, and the proceeds were used to set up a scholarship fund for AIDS patients. I knew that AIDS was the most significant battle that I, and maybe the world, had faced since postwar Poland. But that war was over, and we'd won. With AIDS, the fight was just beginning. While researchers scrambled for funding and raced to find causes and cures, I knew that ultimate victory over this disease depended on more than science.

We were at the start, but I could envision the end. It depended on whether or not we were able to learn the lesson presented by AIDS. In my journal I wrote:

> There is within each of us a potential for goodness beyond our imagining; for giving which seeks no reward; for listening without judgment; for loving unconditionally.

CHAPTER THIRTY-FOUR

Healing Waters

I was still living there, but in the morning light my house looked like I was ready to get out at any moment. The bad smell of burned stuff lingered in the air. And the walls, without my Indian rugs and pictures, were empty. The fire had sucked all the life out of the place, including my own. I had no idea how a good healer like B. could turn into such a dark figure. Until I could get away, I did not want anything to do with him.

Yet as long as I was in close proximity, that was impossible. One morning, shortly after I had returned from a workshop, B. called. His wife had written a book, appropriately called *The Dark Room,* and he wanted me to write a foreword that could be used to publicize it. "Could you have it done by tomorrow morning?" he asked.

As much as I loved my guides, I could not, in good conscience, lend my name to something that had obviously been misused over the past six months. In our last conversation—or should I say confrontation—B. claimed that he could not be held accountable for any of his actions, even if they were improper. "When I'm in a trance, I am not aware of what's happening," he said.

I had no doubt he was a liar, but when it came to actually breaking away, I was torn. I knew that Shanti Nilaya could not survive without my lectures and contributions. After much soul-searching, I called a secret meeting of Shanti Nilaya's most active members, the five women and two men who were actually salaried employees. There I told them everything that was on my mind, including how I feared my life was at risk, the suspicions I had about B. but could not prove, and which entities were real and which were fake.

"Naturally this brings up the whole issue of trust," I said. "It's maddening."

Silence. I told them that at the end of that night's session, I was going to fire B. and his wife and continue Shanti Nilaya without them. I felt relieved just making that decision and sharing it. But then three of the women, the core of my most trusted co-workers, confessed to having been "trained" by the channeler to function as female entities, claiming that he controlled their actions by putting them in trances. No wonder I could never prove Salem or Pedro to be fraudulent—they were real. As for the female entities, they were obviously phony and that explained why they never dealt with me.

I vowed to confront B. the next morning when he came by to pick up the foreword I was supposedly writing. Little did he know I was actually working on a revised ending. The three women agreed to stand behind me as proof. Since nobody knew how B. would react, I asked the two men to hide behind the bushes and listen—just in case. That night I slept little, knowing that I would never see Salem or Pedro again or hear Willie's fine singing. But I had to do what was right.

I rose before dawn, nervous about what was to take place. At the appointed hour, B. arrived. Backed by the three women, I met him on the sun porch. His face was emotionless when I told him that he and his wife were no longer on my payroll; that in fact they were fired. "If you have any questions why, just look at the people here with me and you will know," I said. A hateful look came over his face—his only response. He never uttered a single word. He took the manuscript back up the hill and shortly afterward sold his house and moved to northern California.

I had my freedom, but at a steep price. Through B.'s channeling, many people learned a great deal, but once he started to misuse his gifts, the pain, anguish and agony became intolerable. Much later, when I was able to communicate again with Salem, Pedro and other entities, they acknowledged having been aware of my doubts and constant questioning whether they came from God or the devil. But going through the terrible experience was

244

the only way to learn the ultimate lesson about trust and how to discern and discriminate.

Naturally all was forgiven but not forgotten. It would take seven years before I could listen to the many hours of tape recordings I had made of my spooks' teachings. In hindsight, I would hear explicit warnings about deceit and a terrible split, but they were cryptic and I realized why I had been unable to take concrete action. I had stayed as long as humanly possible. I am convinced I would not have survived if I had stayed with B. any longer. I would continue to have sleepless nights for the rest of my life and ask a million questions, though I knew that I would get the final answers only when I made the transition we call death. I would look forward to it.

Meanwhile, my future was unclear. Even though my house was for sale, I was not going to move until I had someplace to go. So far there wasn't any. The small but dedicated group that remained with Shanti Nilaya worked extremely hard as our organization helped people throughout the world set up similar projects for dying patients, hospices, training centers for health-care professionals, next of kin and bereavement groups. My five-day workshops, given a new urgency by AIDS, were in greater demand than ever before.

If I had wanted to, I could have simply traveled to and from workshops without ever having a home of my own, going from airport to hotel to airport, but that was not me, especially at that point in my life. Knowing I had to slow down, I was wondering how to do that when Raymond Moody, the author of *Life After Life,* whom I had met on occasion, suggested that I check out his farm in the Shenandoahs. It was hard to resist after he described it as "the Switzerland of Virginia." So in mid-1983, after capping a month of travel with a lecture in Washington, D.C., I hired a car to drive me the four and a half hours to Highland County, Virginia.

The driver thought I was nuts. "No matter how much I love this farm, I want you to play the role of my husband and veto my decision," I told him. "I don't want to do something I'll regret later."

But by the time we arrived in Head Waters, the little village about twelve miles from the farm site, the driver, having listened to me gush for hours about the breathtakingly beautiful country-side, reneged on the deal. "Lady, you're gonna buy the land anyway," he explained. "I can tell that it was meant for you."

It seemed that way as I walked the hills and land, up and down, surveying the three hundred acres of pasture and forest. But it was a project. The farmhouse and the barn needed repairs. The tillable land had been neglected. A house would have to be built. Even so, my dream of owning a farm had been fully rekindled. I could easily picture the refurbished farm in my imagination. There would be a healing center, an educational building, some log cabin homes, every kind of animal . . . and privacy. I liked it that Highland County was the least populated area east of the Mississippi.

I actually learned how to go about buying a farm from the elderly farmer who lived at the end of the road. Sort of. Even as I sat across from the head of the local Farm Bureau in Staunton early the next morning, I could not keep myself from telling him all the different ideas I had for my new farm, including a camp for inner-city children, a children's zoo and so on. "Lady, all I need to know is how many head of cattle you have, how many sheep and how many horses and your total acreage," he said.

On July 1, 1983, the next week, I owned the farm. I added life to the farm right away by asking my new neighbors to let their cattle graze on my land and then began extensive reclamation work. From San Diego, I kept close tabs on the progress. In my October newsletter, I wrote: "We have since repainted the farm-house, rebuilt the root cellar, added a section next to the chicken coop . . . and also added a pretty flower and vegetable garden. The result is a full pantry and an already filled root cellar—ready to feed the hungry workshop participants . . ."

By the spring of 1984, there were other signs of renewal. I picked out a site, right beside several towering old-growth oak trees, for the new log cabin that I planned for my own residence. And then the first baby lambs were born, a set of twins and three others—all of them black sheep, which truly made *my* farm.

Construction was underway on the three round structures where I planned to hold workshops when I realized I needed an office for all the organizational needs. Before I rented one in town,

Salem appeared one night and advised me to make a list of everything I needed. I fantasized about a cozy log cabin, with a fireplace, a trout stream running in the front, lots of acreage surrounding it, and then, only because this was a fantasy, I added an airstrip to the list. The airport was so far away, so why not?

The next day the lady at the post office who knew I wanted an office told me an adorable cabin five minutes away from her had just gone up for sale. It was beside the river, she said, and it had a stone fireplace. It sounded perfect. "There's just one problem," she said, already disappointed. Then she didn't want to tell. She begged me to see it first. I refused, and finally managed to persuade her to tell me the one big detraction. "There's a runway in the back," she said. Not only did I gasp; I bought the damn place.

That summer, exactly one year after buying the farm, I said goodbye to Escondido and moved to Head Waters, Virginia, on July 1, 1984. My son Kenneth drove my old Mustang across the country. Fourteen of the fifteen Shanti Nilaya staff members followed me there, helping to continue our important work. Most would leave after a year, unable or unwilling to adopt a lifestyle closer to the earth. My intention was to hit the ground running by finishing the healing center first, but my guides warned me to get my house done first.

I didn't understand why they had said that until a small army of volunteers, answering the plea for help in our newsletter, descended, bringing tools, enthusiasm and special needs. Among forty people, for instance, there might've been thirty-five different diets. One person didn't eat any dairy. Another was macrobiotic. Another didn't eat sugar. Some couldn't eat chicken. Others ate fish. Thank God for my spooks. If I hadn't had the privacy of my own home at night, I would've gone berserk. It took me five years to learn to serve just two kinds of meals—a meat dish and a vegetarian dish.

Slowly, the farm was rehabilitated. I bought tractors and balers. The fields were tilled, reseeded and fertilized. Wells were dug. Of course, the only thing that flowed away seemed to be money. About eight years passed before I broke even, and then only by selling enough sheep, cattle and lumber. But the rewards of living closer to the land by far surpassed the expense.

On the night before Thanksgiving, I was pounding nails

alongside my head construction worker when I got a strong feeling that something very unusual was going to happen, something good. I refused to let him go home and kept him awake all night with coffee and Swiss chocolates—he thought I was nuts. Even so, I promised it would be worthwhile, and sure enough, late that evening, as we sat and talked, the room filled with a warm light. The worker looked at me, as if to say, "What's up?"

"Wait," I said.

Gradually, an image appeared against the far wall. It was immediately apparent who it was. Jesus. He gave his blessings and disappeared. He came back again, left and then returned once more and asked me to name the farm Healing Waters Farm. "It is a new beginning, Isabel."

My witness was incredulous. "Life is full of surprises," I said.

In the morning, we walked outside into the fresh morning air and saw that a gentle snow had fallen, covering the fields, hills and buildings.

It looked like a new beginning.

The move to Healing Waters reenergized me with a sense of mission, though I had no idea what that might be other than settling in. That was enough to start with. One neighbor, Pauline, an angel who was slowed by diabetes, lupus and arthritis, would call the moment I turned on the light after returning home from a trip. It didn't feel like I was home until I heard her warm voice say, "Hello, Elisabeth. Welcome back. Do you mind if I bring something over?" A few minutes later, she was at the door with homemade pudding or apple pie. There were two brothers down the road who were glad to take on any job I gave them.

There was an honesty amid the hardships people suffered in this poor area of the country, people I identified with, who were decidedly more real than the phonies I'd encountered in Southern California, and my own life assumed those same long days, achy muscles and hard-earned rewards. And it might have stayed that way if not for the damn efficiency of the U.S. mail. Efficiency? Yes. I might be the first person ever to complain about that.

When I first arrived, the one-room Head Waters post office was open just one day a week. I warned the sweet woman who ran it that she might have to open more often, since my mail totaled about 15,000 letters a month. "Well, dear, let's see how it goes," she said. After a month, she opened up five days a week, never missing a delivery.

That spring I received a letter that affected my life more than any other. Written on a half sheet of paper, in a heartbreaking simplicity, it said:

Dear Dr. Ross,
　　I have a three-year-old son who has AIDS. I can no longer take care of him. He eats very little and drinks very little. How much would you charge to take care of him?

Similar letters followed. No story illustrated the tragic frustration AIDS patients faced than that of Dawn Place. She was an AIDS-stricken mother in Florida who, in the last painful months of her life, desperately tried to find a place that would agree to care for her daughter, who also had AIDS, after she was dead. More than seventy agencies turned her down, and she died without ever knowing who would care for her child. I got another pathetic letter from a mother in Indiana who asked if I could take care of her AIDS-infected baby. "Nobody wants to touch him," she said.

Though hard to believe, my outrage grew even more when I heard about an AIDS baby in Boston who'd been left in a shoebox to die. Taken in by a hospital, she was put in a crib that was as much a home as a cage is to an animal in the zoo. Hospital workers patted and pinched her daily. But that was it. The child never bonded with anyone. She never got a hug, never cuddled or sat on someone's lap. At two years of age, she didn't know how to crawl, never mind walk, and she wasn't able to speak. It was cruel.

I worked feverishly until I found a marvelous loving couple who agreed to adopt this child. But when they arrived at the hospital, they weren't allowed to see the baby. Administrators gave some excuse about the child being sick. Well, naturally. The baby had AIDS! Eventually, we kidnapped the girl, worked out a settlement after threatening to expose the hospital to the media, and happily the child is now looking foward to becoming a teenager.

249

From then on, I had nightmares of AIDS babies dying without anyone giving them care or love. They stopped only after I heeded the clarion voice of my heart, which instructed me to set up a hospice for AIDS babies on my farm. It wasn't how I'd dreamed of using the farm, but I knew better than to argue with destiny. Before long, I was envisioning a kind of Noah's ark paradise, a place where my AIDS children could romp freely among horses, cows, sheep, peacocks and llamas.

But it turned out much different. On June 2, 1985, while speaking to the graduating class at Mary Baldwin College in Staunton, I casually mentioned my plan to adopt twenty AIDS babies and raise them on five acres that I'd dedicate as a hospice. The students applauded, but my remarks, which were broadcast on local TV and carried in the newspaper, ignited an angry uproar among county residents who, in their fear and ignorance, soon viewed me as the Antichrist trying to bring this deadly disease into their homes.

At first, I was too busy to be aware of the tempest brewing around me. Earlier I had visited a wonderful hospice in San Francisco, where AIDS patients were given compassionate, caring support. It caused me to wonder about AIDS patients in prison, where there was a great deal of sexual abuse and promiscuity and certainly no kind of support system. I called officials in Washington, D.C., alerting them to this epidemic, which was spreading like wildfire, and urging them to prepare for it. They ridiculed my concern. "We don't have a single AIDS patient in prison," they told me.

"You may not know it yet," I argued, "but I'm sure that you have a lot of them."

"No, no, you're right," they replied. "We had four. They were released. The others were all discharged."

I kept making calls, until I spoke to someone who pulled strings and got me into the prison in Vacaville, California. I was told they had no idea how to handle AIDS, so if I was interested in checking out the problem, then by all means go to it. Within twenty-four hours, I was on a plane heading west.

The things I saw inside the prison confirmed my worst fears. There were actually eight inmates dying of AIDS. They suffered

250

without decent care and lived in totally deplorable circumstances, each one isolated in his cell. Only a couple were able to walk and get around; the others were too weak to get out of bed. They told me they didn't have bedpans or portable pots and so were forced to urinate into their drinking cups and empty them out the window.

That was bad enough, but it got worse. One man whose body was covered with cancerous purple Kaposi lesions, begged for radiation treatments. Another inmate's mouth was so covered with a yeast infection that he could barely swallow and I saw him nearly vomit when the guard brought in his lunch—hard-shelled tacos and hot sauce. "I guess they're actually trying to be sadistic," I said, horrified.

The prison's physician was a retired country doctor. My questioning forced him to admit that his knowledge of AIDS was less than the norm, but he made no apologies.

I publicized the sorry conditions I found in that prison through interviews and my book *AIDS: The Ultimate Challenge*. As a project, it became one of my most successful. In December 1986, two of my best California associates, Bob Alexander and Nancy Jaicks, began making weekly support visits to the AIDS prisoners in Vacaville. Their efforts then inspired the U.S. Department of Justice to investigate the living conditions of convicts with AIDS in all prisons. "A start has been made," Bob wrote me optimistically in August 1987.

That's all we needed. A decade later, I went back to Vacaville and saw that what had once been a terribly inhumane situation was completely transformed into a compassionate, enlightened hospice for prisoners with AIDS. They had trained criminals to serve as hospice workers. There was also proper food, medical attention, soothing music, emotional and physical counseling and priests, ministers and rabbis on twenty-four-hour call. I was never so moved in all my life.

For good reason. Even in the grim environment of prison, the tragic suffering of AIDS had brought about generous acts of compassion and caring.

That was an important lesson for anyone who doubted the power of love to make a difference.

PART IV

"THE EAGLE"

CHAPTER THIRTY-FIVE

Service Rendered

✒

While traveling, as I had been for four weeks through Europe, I rarely saw anything but hotels, conference rooms and airports. So there was nothing more spectacularly beautiful than arriving back home. On my first morning back, I drank in the whole lush and lively environment as it awakened— some eighty sheep, cattle, llamas, chickens, turkeys, geese, burros and ducks. The fields had produced an abundance of vegetables. I could imagine no better home than my farm for AIDS-infected children who had no one else to care for them.

There was just one major problem: the people around me did not agree. The phone rang with crank calls. Letters by the boxload awaited me at home. "Take your AIDS babies to some other place," said an anonymous one reflecting popular opinion. "Don't infect us."

Most of the people in the county called themselves good Christians, but they failed to convince me of it. Ever since I had announced my plan to create a hospice for AIDS babies, the people of Highland County had protested against it. They were not particularly well informed about AIDS, and their fears were easily inflamed. While I had been traveling, a construction worker whom I had fired had gone door to door spreading lies about AIDS and asking people to sign a petition opposing me. "Vote no if you don't want this woman to import AIDS into our county," he told people.

He had done a good job. On October 9, 1985, the date of a

town meeting to discuss the matter, people were so outraged they were threatening violence. At that night's meeting, more than half of the county's 2,900 residents filled the tiny Methodist church in Monterey, the county seat. Prior to announcing my plans to adopt AIDS babies, I was greeted warmly and respected as the area's celebrity. But when I walked into the church, people who had once waved at me in town booed and hissed. I knew my chance of winning any of them to my side was already lost.

But even so I got up in front of the tense crowd and described the sort of children I intended to adopt—children between six months and two years old, children "dying of AIDS who have no toys, no love, no sunshine, no hugs, no kisses, no loving environment. They are literally doomed to spend the rest of their lives in those very expensive hospitals." It was as honest and emotional a plea as I could make. Yet I finished to a stony silence.

But I had arranged for more. First the very serious director of the Staunton Heath Department delivered a factual presentation about AIDS, including the specifics of transmission, which should have calmed the fears of any normal thinking human being. Then a woman spoke of how one of her premature twins had contracted AIDS from a tainted blood transfusion, and though the boys shared a crib, bottles and toys, only the infected one died. "His brother has remained negative," she said in a teary voice. Finally a pathologist from Virginia shared his experiences as both a doctor *and* a father who had lost his only son to AIDS.

Unbelievably, each speaker was booed, leaving me outraged and just boiling mad at the ignorance and hatred. I knew the only way that I could have gotten a positive reaction from that crowd would have been to announce my immediate departure from the county. But instead, unwilling to concede defeat, I asked for questions.

Question: "Do you think you are Jesus?"

Answer: "No, I am not Jesus. But I am trying to do what was taught for two thousand years, and that is to love your fellow man, and help them."

Question: "Why don't you set up the center in a place where it will be of the most value immediately? Why put them in this area?"

Answer: "Because I live here, and this is where I work."

Question: "Why didn't you stay where you were at?"

It was close to midnight when the meeting broke up. The point? Nothing. The outcome? Lots of frustration and anger. They hated me. My assistants, the guest speakers and I were escorted out of the church by several policemen, who followed us all the way to my farm. I remarked to my friend that I had no idea the police were so friendly. "Silly, they're not friendly," he said, shaking his head in disbelief. "They're making sure they don't have a lynching tonight."

After that I was an open and easy target. On shopping trips to town, I was called "nigger lover". I received threatening phone calls daily. "You're gonna die just like the AIDS babies you love." The Ku Klux Klan burned crosses on my lawn. Others shot bullets through my windows. Of all the stuff I handled, what annoyed me most were the flat tires I got every time I drove off my property. Living in the boonies, that was a real pain. But obviously someone was sabotaging my truck.

Finally, one night I hid in the farmhouse and spied on the front gate where my truck got all the flats. About two in the morning, I saw six pickup trucks cruise slowly by the gate and toss out pieces of glass and nails. Realizing I had to outsmart them, the following day I dug a hole at the end of my driveway and installed a cattle guard—a metal grid that would allow the sharp debris to fall into the hole—and that put an end to the flats. But it did nothing to help my popularity in Head Waters, or lack of it.

One day, while I was out working, a truck slowed down and the driver yelled out some horrible thing to me. As he sped off, I noticed a bumper sticker on his truck that said, "Jesus Is the Way." Not that way, certainly, and in my frustration, I could not help but call out, "Who are the true Christians around here?"

A year later, I gave up the fight. The forces against me were too strong. Not only was popular opinion against me; the county refused to approve the necessary zoning ordinances. Except for selling the farm, which I was not going to do, I had run out of options, resources and energy. One of the most heartbreaking things I did was walk into the bedroom I had prepared for the children's arrival by filling it with stuffed animals, dolls, handmade

257

quilts and hand-knit sweaters. It looked like a baby store. It seemed all I could do was sit on one of the beds and cry.

But soon I came up with a new plan. If I could not adopt AIDS-infected babies myself, then I would find other people who could do it with much less hassle. I marshaled my considerable resources, including the 25,000 worldwide subscribers to my Shanti Nilaya newsletter, to spread the word. Soon my office resembled a kind of foster agency that matched children to families. One Massachusetts family adopted seven children. Eventually I'd find 350 loving, caring people across the country to adopt AIDS-infected children.

In addition, I heard from people who couldn't adopt children but wanted to help in some way. One elderly woman found a new purpose in life, repairing old dolls she collected at flea markets and sending them to me to give out at Christmas. A Florida attorney offered free legal advice. A Swiss family sent 10,000 francs. A woman proudly told me how she prepared meals once a week for an AIDS patient she met at one of my workshops. Yet another woman wrote that she had overcome her fears and hugged a young man dying of AIDS. It was, she told me, hard to say which one of them benefited most.

The times were marked by violence and hatred, and AIDS was seen as one of the major curses of our time. But I also saw the tremendous good in it. Yes, good. Every one of the thousands of patients I spoke to about their near-death experiences recalled going into the light and being asked, "How much love have you been able to give and receive? How much service have you rendered?" In other words, they were being asked how they had fared in learning the hardest of all of life's lessons: unconditional love.

The AIDS epidemic asked the same question. It generated story after story about people learning to help and love other people. The number of hospices multiplied enormously. I heard of a little boy and his mother taking food to two gay neighbors who could not leave their house. The Names Project memorial quilt is one of the greatest monuments to humanity this country and the world has ever created. When was the last time anyone had heard so many stories like that? Or seen so many examples?

An orderly in one of my workshops told me about a young gay

man who lay dying in his hospital ward. He spent each day in the dark, waiting, aware that his time was running out, and wishing that his father who had kicked him out of the house would come see him before it was too late.

Then one night the orderly notices an older man walking the halls, aimless, nervous and looking forlorn. He's familiar with the people who visit his patients, but he hasn't seen this man before. His intuition tells him it's this guy's father. So when he nears the right room the orderly says, "Your son's in there."

"Not my son," the man replied.

In his gentle, understanding way, the orderly gave the door a slight kick, nudging it open just a crack, and then said, "Here is your son." At that point, the man couldn't help but sneak a quick look at the skeletal patient lying in the dark. After sticking his head inside, he pulled back and said, "No, impossible, that's not my son." But then the patient, in his weakened state, managed to say, "Yes, Dad, it's me. Your son."

The orderly held the door open, and the father slowly walked inside the room. He stood there for a moment, then sat on the bed and hugged his son.

The orderly couldn't recall if he ever let go.

Later that night his son died. But he died at peace and not before letting his father learn the biggest lesson of all.

I had no doubt that one day medical science would discover a cure for this horrible disease. But I hoped not before AIDS cured what ailed us as human beings.

CHAPTER THIRTY-SIX

The Country Doctor

My job was helping people find a more peaceful life, yet there seemed to be no real serenity in my own. The intense fight to adopt AIDS-infected babies exacted a more significant toll than I realized. Then came a hard winter, plus rains and floods that damaged the property. Then there was a drought that ruined a good harvest when we desperately needed one. If that was not enough, I also kept up a full schedule of lectures, workshops, fund-raising activities, house calls and hospital visits.

I ignored warnings from friends that I was driving myself toward serious health problems by taking off on an intensive workshop and lecture tour through Europe. But I rewarded myself at the end by taking two days off to visit my sister Eva in Switzerland. By the time I got there, I was absolutely drained. I looked horrible, in need of a rest, and she pleaded with me to cancel my trip to Montreal and stay longer.

Even though that was impossible, I was determined to make the best of my short visit by enjoying the family party Eva had organized at a nice restaurant. Since a family get-together was a rare event, it was nice and festive, a real treat. "This is what families should do," I said. "They should celebrate while everyone's alive."

"I agree," she said.

"Maybe in future generations people will celebrate when someone graduates and not make such a big sad absurdity out of dying," I continued. "If anything, people should mourn when someone's born and has to start the whole nonsense of living all over again."

Twenty-four hours later, while preparing for bed, I told my sister not to fuss the next morning—that I'd drink some coffee, smoke a cigarette and then take off for the airport. In the morning my alarm went off, and by the time I got myself downstairs I saw that not only had Eva ignored me, she had gotten out her fancy white tablecloth and fashioned a center-piece of beautiful fresh flowers. I sat down for coffee and as I got ready to scold her for doing too much, the thing everyone feared most happened.

All of the stress and garbage, all of the travel, the coffee, cigarettes and chocolate—all of it—suddenly caught up with me. I was seized by an odd sinking sensation. My body got weak. Everything began swirling around me. I lost consciousness of my sister and could not move. Yet I knew exactly what was happening.

I was dying.

I knew it instantly. After helping so many through their final moments, my own death had finally agreed to arrive. The comments I had made to my sister the previous night at the restaurant now seemed prophetic. At least I was going out with a celebration. I also pictured the farm, the fields that were full of vegetables that would need canning, the cows, pigs, sheep, and the new baby animals. Then I looked at Eva, who sat directly across from me. She had helped me so much with my work in Europe and on the farm. I wanted to give her something before I died.

There seemed to be no way to do that, since I did not know how I was dying. If, for instance, it was a coronary, I could go in an instant. Then I got an idea.

"Eva, I'm dying," I said. "And I want to give you a goodbye present. I'm going to share with you what it really feels like to die from the patient's point of view. It's the best gift I can give, because nobody ever talks while they experience it."

I did not wait—or even notice, for that matter—for her to react before I launched into a detailed commentary of exactly what was happening to me. "It's starting in my toes," I said. "They feel like they are in hot water. Numbing. Soothing." To me, my voice sounded like it was going as fast as the announcer's at a horse race. "It's moving up my body—my legs. Now past my waist.

"I am not scared. It's just as I thought. It's a pleasure. It's really a pleasurable feeling."

I knocked myself out to keep pace with what I was experiencing.

"I'm outside my body," I continued. "No regrets. Tell Kenneth and Barbara goodbye.

"Just love."

At that point, I had a second or two left. I felt as if I were on a ski slope, preparing to jump over the edge. Ahead was the bright light. I put my arms out in an angle that would enable me to fly straight into the center of the light. I remember crouching down in a racing position to gain momentum and control. I was completely aware that the final glorious moment had arrived and enjoying every revelatory second. "I am about to graduate," I said to my sister. Then I stared at the light straight in front of me, felt it draw me closer and opened my arms wide. "Here I come!" I screamed.

When I woke up again I was lying flat across the table in Eva's kitchen. My sister's fancy white tablecloth was covered with spilled coffee. Her beautiful flower arrangement was scattered all over the place. Even worse, Eva was a wreck. Panicked out of her mind, she held me while trying to figure out what to do. She apologized for not calling an ambulance. "Don't be a jerk," I said. "You don't have to call them. Obviously I didn't take off. I'm stuck here again."

Eva insisted on doing something, so I made her take me to the airport, even though it was against her better judgment. "To hell with judgment," I scoffed. On the way, however, I asked her to tell me about the gift I'd given her, my account of what it was like to die. That got me a weird look. I could tell that she wondered if I was already airborne. All she heard me say was "I'm dying," and then "Here I come." Everything between was a complete blank, except for the crashing sound of dishes flying as I hit the table.

Three days later I diagnosed the problem as a slight fibrillation of my heart, maybe something else but nothing serious. I pronounced myself fine. But I wasn't fine. The drought-plagued summer of 1988 was hard. During record heat waves, I supervised completion of the center's round houses, popped over to Europe and celebrated my sixty-second birthday by throwing a party for families who had adopted AIDS-infected babies. By the end of July, I was dragging more than usual.

I ignored the fatigue. Then, on August 6, I was driving with Ann, a doctor friend visiting from Australia, and my former helper, Charlotte, a nurse, down a steep hill above the farm. Suddenly, I felt a contraction in my head, a painful stitch that sent a kind of electrical shudder down my right side. I grabbed my head with my left hand and pressed down hard. Gradually, my right side got weaker and then grew numb. I turned to Ann, who was in the front seat, and calmly said, "I just had a stroke."

None of us knew what to think right then. Were we scared? Did any of us panic? No. You couldn't have found three more capable, coolheaded women. Somehow I managed to steer the truck back to the farmhouse and put on the brake. "How are you, Elisabeth?" they asked. I honestly didn't know. By then, I couldn't speak clearly anymore. My tongue didn't work properly, my mouth hung there as if the parts had just worn out and my right arm didn't follow orders.

"We have to get her to the hospital," Ann said.

"Baloney," I managed to say. "What can they do for a stroke? They do nothing except watch."

But, aware that I needed at least a basic checkup, I let them take me to the University of Virginia's Medical Center. Instead of cooking dinner that night, I sat in the emergency room. I was the only one there dying for a cup of coffee and a cigarette. The best they gave me was a doctor who refused to admit me unless I stopped smoking. "No!" I snapped. He folded his arms, a real big shot making a point. I had no idea that he was chief of the stroke unit. Nor did I care. "This is my life," I said.

Meanwhile, a young doctor, amused by the tussle, mentioned that a university bigwig's wife, recently admitted to the stroke unit, had used her pull to get a private room where she could smoke. "Ask if she minds a roommate," I said. She was delighted to have the company. The minute the door shut, my roommate, an intelligent and very amusing seventy-one-year-old woman, and I lit our cigarettes. We acted like two naughty teenagers. Whenever I heard footsteps, I gave a signal and we snuffed out our cigarettes.

Admittedly not an easy patient, I nevertheless got bad treatment. No one took a decent case history. No one did a thorough workup. Nurses woke me up every hour through the night by shining a flashlight directly in my eyes. "Are you sleeping?" they asked. "Not anymore," I grumbled. On my final night in the hospital, I asked the nurse if she could wake me up by playing music. "We can't do that," the nurse said. "How about whistling or singing?" I suggested. "We can't do that either," she answered.

That's all I ever heard: "We can't do that."

Finally I had enough. At eight o'clock on my third morning there, I limped to the nursing station—with my roommate right behind me—and checked myself out. "You can't do that," they told me.

"Wanna bet?" I said.

"But you can't."

"I'm a doctor," I said.

"No, you're a patient."

"Patients have rights too," I said. "I'll sign the papers."

I recuperated better and faster at home than I would've in the hospital. I slept well and ate good food. I created my own rehabilitation program. Every day I got myself dressed and climbed the large hill behind my farm. It was the wilderness, with bears and snakes lurking behind trees and rocks. I started by crawling up the path on my hands and knees, slowly and painfully. By the end of the first week, I was on my feet again, leaning on a cane but regaining my strength. On each hike, I sang at the top of my voice, a great exercise, and with my dreadful off-key warbling it was also a surefire method of protection from wild animals.

After four weeks—despite my doctor's pessimism—I was able to walk and talk again. Fortunately, it had been a "little" stroke, and I resumed gardening, farming, writing, cooking and traveling, everything I had done before. There was no mistaking the message to slow down. But how about mellowing out? Not likely, as evidenced by the lecture I gave in October to doctors at the hospital that I'd checked myself out of two months earlier. "You cured me," I exclaimed in jest. "In two days, you people cured me from ever wanting to be hospitalized unless it is a red-hot emergency!"

In the summer of 1989, I enjoyed my finest harvest ever. I'd owned the farm for five years, worked it for four and savored the fruits and vegetables of my hard labor. There was truth in the biblical statement: You reap what you sow. It was early fall, prime color season, before I finished all the canning and preserving chores and started germinating the next year's seedlings in the greenhouse. Living closer to the land, I appreciated our dependency on Mother Earth more than ever and found myself paying more attention to Hopi prophecies and the Book of Revelation.

I worried about the future of the world. As portrayed in newspapers and on CNN, it looked scary. I gave credence to people who warned that the planet would soon be rocked by catastrophic events. My own journals were filled with thoughts and ideas intended to prevent that kind of pain and suffering. "If we view ALL living things as a gift of God, created for our pleasure and enjoyment, to love and respect, to treasure and to guard for our next generations, and look after our own self with the same loving care—the future will be something NOT TO BE FEARED, but treasured."

Unfortunately, all those journals would be destroyed. But a few other entries come to mind:

- Our todays depend on our yesterdays and our tomorrows depend on our todays.
- Have you loved yourself today?
- Have you admired and thanked the flowers, treasured the birds or gazed up at the mountains and felt a sense of awe?

There were days when I felt my age, when my body ached and reminded me of just what an impatient person I was. But when I pondered life's big questions in my workshops, I felt as young and vital and hopeful as I did when I was a country doctor making my first house call more than forty years earlier. The best medicine of all is the simplest medicine. "Let's all learn self-love, self-forgiveness, compassion and understanding," I took to saying at the end of workshops. It was a summary of all my knowledge and experience. "Then we'll be able to give those gifts to others. By healing the person, we can heal Mother Earth."

CHAPTER THIRTY-SEVEN

Graduation

After seven years of work, struggle and tears, I was happy to have good reason to celebrate. On a brilliant July afternoon in 1990, I oversaw the official grand opening festivities dedicating the Elisabeth Kübler-Ross Center—an event that truly began twenty years earlier when I felt the first impulse to own a farm. Though the facilities were regularly used for workshops, all the construction was finally completed.

As I stood in the center and gazed at the buildings, the cabins, my Swiss flag flying outside the center, a part of me could not believe the sight. The dream had endured my divorce, gained momentum when I started Shanti Nilaya in San Diego and miraculously survived both my crisis of faith with B. and my battle with the local population, who would have preferred that this so-called AIDS-loving old lady take the first bus out of town.

After the blessing, touchingly given by my longtime friend Mwalimu Imara, there was gospel and country music and enough homemade food to feed the five hundred friends who had come from as far away as Alaska and New Zealand. There was also much catching up with family members and former patients. It was a great day that renewed my faith in destiny. Alas, not everyone whose life had touched my own was able to celebrate in person, but only two months earlier I received an unforgettable reminder of all of them and why I could consider myself truly blessed. It read:

Dear Elisabeth:

Today is Mother's Day and I have more hope on this day than I have had in four years! I just got back yesterday from the Life, Death and Transition workshop in Virginia and I had to write and tell you how it affected me.

Three and a half years ago, my six-year-old daughter, Katie, died of a brain tumor. Shortly afterwards, my sister sent me a copy of the Dougy Book and the words you shared in that booklet touched me deeply. The message of the caterpillar and the butterfly continue to bring hope and it was so important to hear the message from you last Thursday. Thanks for being there to share yourself with us.

I cannot begin to tell you about all of the gifts I received from that week but I do want to share some of the gifts I received from my daughter's life and death. Thanks to you, I understand more about my daughter's life and death. We shared a special bond all through her life but most clearly through her illness and death. She taught me much as she died and she continues to be my teacher.

Katie died in 1986 after a nine-month battle with a malignant brain stem tumor. After five months, she lost her ability to walk and to talk but not to communicate. People would be so confused when they would see her in a semi-coma-like state and I would tell them that we talked all the time. I certainly continued to talk with her and she with me. We insisted she be allowed to die at home and even brought her to the beach with my family two weeks before her death. It was a very important time for all of us, including several young nieces and nephews who learned much about life and death during the week. I know they will long remember how they helped take care of her.

A week after we returned home, she died. That day began as usual with giving her medications and food, bathing her and talking to her. That morning as her ten-year-old sister left for school, Katie made some sounds (something she hadn't done for months) and I commented that she was saying "Goodbye" to Jenny before she went to school. I noticed she looked very tired and I promised I wouldn't move her any more that day. I talked to her and told her not to be afraid, that I was with her and that she would be OK. I said that she did not have to hold on for me and that when she died she would be safe and surrounded with people who loved her, like her grandfather who had died two years previously. I told her that we would miss her a lot but that we would be OK. Then I sat with her in the living room. Later that afternoon, Jenny came home, said hi to Katie and went into the other room to begin homework. Something told me to go over to Katie and I started cleaning her feeding tube, which was leaking. As I looked up at her, her lips turned white. She took two breaths and stopped. I talked to her and she blinked her eyes twice and was gone. I knew that there was nothing to do except hold her and so I did. I felt sad but very peaceful. I never considered CPR, which I knew how to do. Thanks to you, I understand why. I knew her life ended when it ended and that she had learned all she came to learn and taught all she came to teach. Much of my time now is spent in trying to understand how much she did teach as she lived and as she died.

Immediately after her death and since, I began to experience a surge of energy and I wanted to write. I wrote for several days and I continue to be amazed at the energy and the messages I get. Immediately after her death, I was filled with the message that my life has a mission, that reaching out and giving to others is what life is all about. "Katie will live forever as we all will. The essence of what is most valuable must be shared with others. Loving, sharing, enriching others' lives, touching and being touched—can anything else measure up to these moments?"

And so since Katie's death, I have embarked on a new life—beginning a degree in counseling which I completed in December, working with people with AIDS . . . and understanding more and more about my spiritual bonds with Katie and God.

I would also like to share a dream I had several months after Katie's death. This dream had a very real quality to it and I knew when I awoke it was significant. Your discussion last Thursday added some meaning to it for me:

I approached a stream that separated me from another place. I knew that I had to go there. I saw a narrow footbridge that crossed a stream. My husband was with me and walked behind for a while and then I had to carry him across the bridge. When we reached the other side, we entered a lodge. Inside were many children wearing tags with their names and pictures. We found Katie and we knew that these were all children who had died and that we would be allowed to visit for a while. We went over to Katie and I asked if I could hold her. She said, "Yes, we can play for a while but I cannot leave with you." I said that I knew that. We visited and played for a while and then we had to go.

I awoke with a clear feeling that I had been with Katie that night. Now I know I had.

Love, M.P.

Manny's Signal

There was no other way to look at it: I was surrounded by murderers, people who had committed some of the worst crimes against human beings that I had ever heard of. There was no escape either. We were all locked behind bars in a maximum-security prison in Edinburgh, Scotland. And I was asking them for a confession—not of whatever gruesome crime they had committed. No, I wanted something far more troubling, far more painful. I wanted them to admit the inner pain that had caused them to murder.

Sure, it was a novel approach to reform, but I believed that even a life sentence had no chance of helping a murderer change unless the trauma that had motivated such a vicious crime was externalized. It was the same theory behind my workshops. In 1991, I proposed holding one behind bars to numerous prisons, including U.S. facilities, and only the Scottish prison agreed to my novel terms—that half the workshop participants be prisoners and the other half prison staffers.

Would it work? Based on experience, there was no question. For an entire week, all of us lived in the prison, ate the same food, slept on the same hard beds, showered in the same cold stalls (except for me—I would rather stink to death than freeze) and got locked up together at night. By the end of the first day, after most of the men explained what misdeeds got them incarcerated, tears flowed out of even the hardest prisoner. During the rest of the week, most revealed stories of childhoods that had been scarred by sexual and emotional abuse.

But the prisoners were not the only ones sharing. After the prison warden, a slight woman, relived an intimate problem from her youth in front of the prisoners and guards, the group was bonded by an emotional closeness. Despite their differences, there was suddenly real compassion, empathy and love for each other. By week's end, they recognized what I had long ago discovered—that everyone, like true brothers and sisters, is bonded by pain and exists solely to endure hardship and grow.

While the inmates got the kind of peace that would allow them to live whole lives even behind bars, I was rewarded with the best Swiss meal I ever had abroad and a touching goodbye tune from a Scottish bagpiper, maybe the only time those prisoners were going to hear music like that inside those walls. Although such workshops were incredibly productive, they were rare. My hope was that they would inspire similar programs in overcrowded U.S. prisons where no attention is given to healing.

People would scoff at such goals and called them unrealistic, yet there were plenty of examples of goals that seemed even more impossible, except for the fact that people had committed themselves to making a change. There was no better example than South Africa, where the old repressive system of apartheid was in the process of being replaced by a multiracial democracy.

For years, I had declined offers to hold workshops in South Africa unless I could be guaranteed a mix of black and white participants. Finally, in 1992, two years after African National Congress leader Nelson Mandela had been released from prison, I was promised a racial mix under one roof, and so I agreed to go. Although not exactly following Albert Schweitzer, who had inspired me to become a doctor fifty-five years earlier, I was still fulfilling a lifelong dream.

That workshop, which was an enormous success in forging an understanding of humanity based on people's similarities rather than differences, marked a major achievement. At sixty-six years old, I had conducted workshops on every continent in the world. Afterward I marched in a political rally supporting a peaceful transition to a multiracial government. But it did not matter whether I was in Johannesburg or Chicago, because all destiny leads down the same path—growth, love and service. Being there just reinforced my sense of having already arrived.

But then came a sad matter, one of departure. That fall, Manny, who had survived a triple bypass operation, was greatly weakened when his heart began to fail. Fearing he could not hold up against another harsh Chicago winter when his condition, at best, was iffy, he spent the winters in Scottsdale, Arizona, where the climate was acceptable. In October, he moved into a friend's house. There he was very happy. Long past any grudge about the way our marriage ended, I dropped by whenever I could and filled his fridge with home-cooked meals. Manny sure loved to eat my Swiss meals. He got great care.

I could not say as much for the few weeks Manny had to spend in the hospital after his kidneys began to fail. Even though he was weakening, his mood improved when we brought him back home. Just a few short days before he died, I had to fly to Los Angeles for a conference on hospices. Knowing dying patients have the greatest insight into how much time is actually left, I suggested sticking around, but Manny said that he wanted some private time with other family members. "Fine, I'll go," I said. "Then I'll fly right back in the next few days."

A half hour before leaving for the airport, I remembered the deal I wanted to make with Manny in case he died while I was in California. If all my research about life after death was correct, I wanted him to send me a signal after he died. If it was not valid, then he would not do anything and I would continue my research. Manny procrastinated. "What kind of signal?" he asked. "Something far out," I said. "I don't know exactly, but something that I'll know could only be from you." He was tired and not in the mood. "I'm not leaving until you shake hands," I warned. At the last minute, he agreed and I left in good spirits. It was the last time I saw him alive.

Later that afternoon Kenneth took Manny to the grocery store. It was his first trip outside after being in the hospital for three weeks. On the way home, Manny stopped at the florist and bought a dozen long-stemmed red roses for Barbara to have on her birthday the following day. Then Kenneth brought Manny back to the condo, where he took a nap while Kenneth put the groceries away and then went back to his house.

An hour later, Kenneth returned to make dinner and found Manny passed away in bed. He had died during his afternoon nap.

When I got back to my hotel room late that night I saw the message light on the telephone blinking. Apparently Kenneth had tried to get word to me about Manny much earlier, but we were not able to get in touch until midnight. Meanwhile, Kenneth had called Barbara in Seattle after she got home from work to break the news, and they spent the evening on the phone. The next day, after making more calls to family, Barbara decided to take her dog for a walk. Returning to the house, she came upon the dozen roses Manny had sent her on the doorstep, in the snow that had been falling all morning.

I had no idea about the arrival of the flowers until Manny's funeral in Chicago. I had made my peace with Manny and was happy that he no longer had to suffer. As we stood around the gravesite, it started to snow heavily. I noticed dozens of roses were strewn on the ground around the gravesite and could not stand seeing them go to waste lying there in the snow. So I picked up those gorgeous roses and handed them out to Manny's friends, the people who were genuinely distraught. I gave each person a rose. The last one I gave to Barbara because she was a papa's girl. I remembered the conversation I'd had with Manny when she was about ten years old. We'd been having one of those discussions about my theories of life after death, and he turned to Barbara and said, "Okay, if what your mother says is true, then the first snowfall after I die, there'll be red roses blooming in the snow." Over the years, this wager had become a kind of family joke, but now it was truth.

I was bowled over with joy, and my smile showed it. I looked upward. The gray sky was full of swirling snow that looked to me like celebratory confetti. Manny was up there. Ah, the two of them, my two greatest skeptics. Now they were laughing together. And so was I.

"Thanks," I said, looking up at Manny. "Thanks for confirming it."

The Butterfly

As an expert in dealing with loss, I not only knew the different stages a person goes through after one, I had defined them. Anger. Denial. Bargaining. Depression. Acceptance. On that chilly October night in 1994 when I returned from Baltimore and found my beloved house engulfed by flames, I went through each stage. I was surprised at how quickly I accepted the news. "What can I do about it now?" I said to Kenneth.

After twelve hours, the house still burned as intensely as when I had first driven by the "Healing Waters" signpost the previous midnight and noticed how the black sky was smudged with an eerie orange glow. By then, I had counted my blessings, which included how lucky I was not to have had twenty AIDS babies at risk by living there. I was also unharmed. The loss of possessions was another matter that was beyond my own life. Photo albums and diaries my father had kept were destroyed. So was all my furniture, appliances and clothing. And the journal I had kept of my trip to Poland, which had changed my life. Pictures I took at Maidanek. I also lost twenty-five journals in which I had meticulously recorded all of the conversations I had with Salem and Pedro. Plus hundreds of thousands of pages of documentation, notes and research were gone. All the photographs I had taken of my spooks were destroyed. Countless photographs, books, letters—nothing but ash.

Later that day the brunt of the disaster hit me and I went into a kind of shock. I had lost everything. Until bedtime, I sat, smoked and was unable to do anything beyond that. On the second morning, I climbed out of it. I woke up much better, sober and realistic. What are you going to do? Give up? No. "This is an opportunity to grow," I reminded myself. "You will not grow if everything is perfect. But pain is a gift with its own purpose."

And that purpose was? A chance to rebuild? After surveying the damage, I told Kenneth that was my plan. I was going to rebuild. Right over the ashes. "It's a blessing," I declared. "I don't have to pack anymore. I'm free. Once I've rebuilt, I can spend half the year in Africa and half here."

He had no doubt that I was not in my right mind.

"You aren't rebuilding," he said emphatically. "Next time they'll shoot you."

"Yes, they probably will," I said. "That will be their problem."

My son saw it as his problem too. For the next three days, he listened to me muse on the future while we bunked in the farmhouse. One afternoon he drove into town, ostensibly to pick up a new supply of basics like underwear, socks and jeans for me. Instead he returned with fire alarms, smoke detectors, fire extinguishers and security devices—something for every possible kind of emergency. But that did not alleviate his concern for me. Kenneth did not want me to live there anymore by myself, period.

I had no idea that he was up to something sneaky when he drove me into town for a lobster dinner, one of the few things I would never turn down. But rather than going to a restaurant, we ended up on an airplane bound for Phoenix. Kenneth had moved to Scottsdale to be closer to his father, and now I was following. "We'll find you a house of your own," he said. I didn't protest too much. I had nothing to pack. No clothes, no furniture, no books, no pictures. No house, for that matter. There was really nothing left to keep me in Virginia. Why not move on?

I simply said yes to the pain and it disappeared.

In the river of tears, make time your friend.

A few months later a man in a Monterey bar would confess that he had "gotten rid of the AIDS lady." Even so, local authorities refused to press any charges. The Highland County police told me that they did not have enough evidence. I was not up to fighting. And as for the farm itself? Despite the money and sweat I had put into it, I simply gave the center with the workshop site to a group that worked with abused and troubled teenagers.

That is the great thing about property. I had my chance there. Now it was time for others to try to make the land work for them.

I moved to Scottsdale and found an adobe house in the middle of the desert. There was nothing around me. At night, I sat in the hot tub, listened to the coyotes howl and gazed up at the millions of stars in the galaxy. You could sense the infinity of time. The mornings had a similiar feel—deceptively quiet and still. The rocks hid snakes and rabbits and birds nested in tall cacti. The desert could be both serene and dangerous.

On May 13, 1995, the night before Mother's Day, I had told my houseguest, my German publisher, that I was enjoying the opportunity for reflection that the desert provided. Early the next morning, I heard the phone ring, opened one eye and saw that it was seven o'clock. No one I knew would dare call me at that hour. Maybe it was for my houseguest, someone from Europe. When I tried leaning over to answer it, I knew something was wrong. My body did not move. Would not move. The phone continued to ring. My brain issued the order to move but my body would not obey.

Then I realized the problem. "You have had another stroke," I told myself. "This time it's a massive one."

After the phone went unanswered, I figured that my publisher had gone for a long morning walk. That left me by myself. From what I could discern, the stroke had definitely caused some paralysis, but it appeared to be confined mostly to the left side. Even though I had no strength, I could still move my right arm and leg a bit. I decided to get myself out of bed and into the hallway where I could yell for help. It took close to an hour for me to inch myself onto the floor. I was like a piece of slow-melting cheese. All I thought about was not falling, since I did not want to break my hip. That would have been too much on top of the stroke.

Once on the floor, I spent another hour getting to the door, which I could not open because the doorknob was too high. More time was spent using my nose and chin to painfully pry it open. When I was finally able to stick my head into the hallway I heard my publisher out in the garden, too far away for him to hear my weak voice. After perhaps another thirty minutes, he came in and heard me calling out for help. He drove me to Kenneth's house, where my son and I argued about whether or not I'd go to the hospital. I did not want to. "You can smoke when you get out," he said.

As soon as Kenneth agreed that, no matter what, I could leave the hospital after twenty-four hours, I permitted him to check me into a local hospital. Even then, although paralyzed on my left side, I was reluctant, difficult, complaining and craving a cigarette. Not your ideal patient. They put me through CAT scans, an MRI and all the basic tests, which confirmed what I already knew—that I had suffered a brain stem stroke.

As far as I was concerned, that was nothing compared with the suffering caused by present-day health care. It started in the hospital with an unfriendly nurse and then continued with downright incompetence. On my first afternoon there, a nurse tried straightening out my left arm, which was frozen into a crooked position and so painful I could not even stand air blowing against it. When she grabbed it, I gave her a karate chop with my good right arm, causing her to get two other nurses to hold me down.

"Watch out, she's combative," the first nurse said to the others.

She only knew the half of it, since I checked out the following day. There was no way I was going to put up with that kind of treatment. Unfortunately, a week later, I returned to the hospital with a urinary tract infection from lying still all the time and not drinking enough. Because I had to urinate every half hour, I was forced to rely on the nurses to get me on the commode. On my second night, the door to my room shut, my call button fell to the floor and they completely forgot about me.

It was hot and the air-conditioning was broken. My bladder was ready to burst. It was not a good night. Then I saw my teacup on the night table. It was like a gift from heaven. I used it to relieve myself.

The next morning a nurse came in fresh as a daisy, a smile on her face. "How are you this morning, dear?" she asked. I looked at her with the warmth of a rusty nail. "What's this?" she said, looking in my teacup.

"That's my urine," I said. "No one came in to check on me all night."

"Oh," she said without apologizing, and walked out.

Home care was little better. For the first time in my life, I was on Medicare and it taught me an awful lot—not much of it good. I was assigned a doctor I did not know. This one happened to be a well-known neurologist. Kenneth pushed my wheelchair into his office.

"How are you?" he asked.

"Paralyzed," I said.

Rather than take my blood pressure or vital signs, the doctor asked what books I had written since my first one and then implied that he would appreciate a copy of my latest, preferably autographed. I wanted to change doctors, but Medicare was against it. A month later, though, I had trouble breathing and needed help. My excellent physical therapist called my doctor three times without getting a response. Finally I called myself. His secretary answered and sadly announced the doctor was much too busy. "But you can ask me any question," she chirped pleasantly.

"If I wanted a receptionist, I'd call one," I said. "But I want a doctor."

That was the end of him. His replacement was a wonderful doctor friend of mine, Gladys McGarrey. She took good care of me. She really cared. She made house calls, even on weekends, and she notified me if she was going out of town. She listened to me. She was what I expected from a physician.

The bureaucracy of the health-care system lived down to my expectations. I was assigned social workers who had no intention of doing any work. One woman ignored me when I asked a question about what my insurance covered. "Your son can take care of that," she said. Then there was the seemingly small matter of a seat cushion. A nurse had ordered me a cushion for my tailbone, which ached from sitting fifteen hours a day. When it was delivered I saw that Medicare had been charged $400 for this thing that wasn't worth more than $20. I mailed it back.

A few days later, the company called and told me that I was not allowed to mail the cushion back. It had to be picked up personally by the delivery service. They were sending the damn cushion back. "Fine, send it back," I said incredulously. "I'll be sitting on it."

There was nothing funny about health care. Two months after my stroke, though I continued to be in pain and suffer from paralysis, my physical therapist said that my insurance company had pulled the plug on further treatment. "Dr. Ross, I'm sorry but I won't be coming anymore," she said. "They won't pay for it."

Could any phrase be scarier in terms of a person's health? All my sensibilities as a physician were mortally offended. After all, I had been called into medicine. I had felt honored to treat war victims. I had cared for people considered hopeless. I had dedicated my entire career to teaching doctors and nurses to be more caring and compassionate. In thirty-five years, I had never charged a single patient.

Now I was told, "They won't pay for it."

Was this modern medical care? The decision made by somebody in an office who'd never seen the patient. Had paperwork replaced concern for people?

As far as I am concerned, the values are all out of whack.

Today's medicine is complex and research is costly, but the heads of big insurance companies and HMOs are making millions of dollars in annual salaries. At the same time, AIDS patients are unable to afford life-prolonging drugs. Cancer patients are denied treatment because it is called "experimental." Emergency rooms are being closed. Why is this tolerated? How can anyone be denied hope? Or denied care?

Once upon a time, medicine was about healing, not management. It must adopt that mission again. Doctors, nurses and researchers must recognize that they are the heart of humanity, just as clergymen are its soul. They need to make helping their fellow man—whether rich or poor, whether black, white, yellow or brown—their highest priority. Trust me, as someone who has been paid in "blessed Polish soil," there is no greater reward.

In life after death, everyone faces the same question. *How much service have you rendered? What have you done to help?*

If you wait until then to answer, it will be too late.

282

*   *   *

Death itself is a wonderful and positive experience, but the process of dying, when it is prolonged like mine, is a nightmare. It saps all your faculties, especially patience, endurance and equanimity. Throughout 1996, I struggled with the constant pain and limitations of my paralysis. I am dependent on twenty-four-hour care. If the doorbell rings, I cannot get it. And privacy? That is a thing of the past. After fifteen years of total independence, it is a difficult lesson to learn. People come in, they go out. Sometimes my house is like Grand Central Station. Other times it is too quiet.

What kind of life is this? A miserable one.

By January 1997, the time of this writing, I can honestly say that I am anxious to graduate. I am very weak, in constant pain and totally dependent. According to my Cosmic Consciousness, I know that if I would stop being bitter, angry and resentful of my condition and just say yes to this kind of "end of my life," then I could take off and live in a better place and have a better life. But since I am very stubborn and defiant, I have to learn my final lessons the hard way. Just like everyone else.

Even with all my suffering I am still opposed to Kevorkian, who takes people's lives prematurely simply because they are in pain or are uncomfortable. He does not understand that he deprives people of whatever last lessons they have to learn before they can graduate. Right now I am learning patience and submission. As difficult as those lessons are, I know that the Highest of the High has a plan. I know that He has a time that will be right for me to leave my body the way a butterfly leaves its cocoon.

Our only purpose in life is growth. There are no accidents.

CHAPTER FORTY

On Life and Living

It is just like me to have already planned what will happen. My family and friends will arrive from all parts of the world, wend their way through the desert until they come upon a tiny white sign planted in a dirt road that says *Elisabeth,* and then drive until they reach the Indian tepee and the Swiss flag that stands high above my Scottsdale home. Some will be grieving. Others will know how relieved and happy I finally am. They will eat, trade stories, laugh, cry and at some point release dozens of helium-filled balloons that look like E.T. into the blue sky. Of course, I will be dead.

But why not throw a going-away party? Why not celebrate? At seventy-one years old, I can say that I have truly lived. After starting out as a "two-pound nothing" who was not expected to survive, I spent most of my life battling the Goliath-sized forces of ignorance and fear. Anyone familiar with my work knows that I believe death can be one of life's greatest experiences. Anyone who knows me personally can testify to how impatiently I have been awaiting the transition from the pain and struggle of this world to an existence of complete and overwhelming love.

It has not come easily, this final lesson of patience. For the past two years, I have—thanks to a series of strokes—been totally dependent on others for the most basic care. Every day is spent struggling to get from bed to a chair to the bathroom and then back again. My only wish has been to leave my body, like a butterfly shedding its cocoon, and finally merge with the great light. My spooks have reiterated the importance of making time my friend. I know that the day that will end my life in this form, in this body, will be the day when I have learned that kind of acceptance.

The only benefit of making such a slow approach to life's final passage has been the time it offers for contemplation. I suppose it is appropriate that after counseling so many dying patients I should have time to reflect on death now that the one I face is my own. There is a poetry to it, a slight tension, like a pause in a courtroom drama where the defendant is given the chance to confess. Fortunately, I have nothing new to admit. My death will come to me like a warm embrace. As I have long said, life in a physical body is a very short span of one's total existence.

When we have passed the tests we were sent to Earth to learn, we are allowed to graduate. We are allowed to shed our body, which imprisons our soul the way a cocoon encloses the future butterfly, and when the time is right we can let go of it. Then we will be free of pain, free of fears and free of worries . . . free as a beautiful butterfly returning home to God . . . which is a place where we are never alone, where we continue to grow and to sing and to dance, where we are with those we loved, and where we are surrounded with more love than we can ever imagine.

Thankfully, I have reached a level where I no longer have to come back to learn any more lessons, but sadly I am not comfortable with the world I am departing for the last time. The whole planet is in trouble. This is a very tenuous time in history. Earth has been abused for too long without regard for any serious consequences. Mankind has wreaked havoc with the bounty of God's garden. Weapons, greed, materialism, destructiveness. They have become the catechism of life, the mantra of generations whose meditations on the meaning of life have gone dangerously awry.

I believe Earth will soon correct these misdeeds. Because of what mankind has done, there will be tremendous earthquakes, floods, volcanic eruptions and other natural disasters on a scale never before witnessed. Because of what mankind has forgotten, there will be enormous casualties suffered. I know this. My spooks have told me to expect upheavals and seizures of biblical proportions. How else can people be awakened? What other way is there to teach respect for nature and the necessity of spirituality?

Just as my eyes have seen the future, my heart goes out to those who are left behind. Do not be afraid. There is no cause for it, if you remember that death does not exist. Instead know your own self and view life as a challenge where the hardest choices are the highest ones, the ones that will resonate with righteousness and provide the strength and insight of Him, the Highest of the High. *The greatest gift God has given us is free choice.* There are no accidents. Everything in life happens for a positive reason. *Should you shield the canyons from the windstorms, you would never see the beauty of their carvings.*

As I pass from this world to the next, I know that heaven or hell is determined by the way people live their lives in the present. *The sole purpose of life is to grow. The ultimate lesson is learning how to love and be loved unconditionally.* There are millions of people on Earth who are starving. There are millions who are homeless. There are millions who have AIDS. There are millions of people who have been abused. There are millions of people who struggle with disabilities. Every day someone new cries out for understanding and compassion. Listen to the sound. Hear the call as if it was beautiful music. I can assure you that the greatest rewards in your whole life will come from opening your heart to those in need. The greatest blessings always come from helping.

I truly believe that my truth is a universal one—above all religions, economics, race and color—shared by the common experience of life.

All people come from the same source and return to the same source.

We must all learn to love and be loved unconditionally.

All the hardships that come to you in life, all the tribulations and nightmares, all the things you see as punishments from God, are in reality like gifts. They are an opportunity to grow, which is the sole purpose of life.

You cannot heal the world without healing yourself first.

If you are ready for spiritual experiences and you are not afraid, you will have them yourself. You do not need a guru or a Baba to tell you how to do it.

All of us, when we were born from the source, which I call

God, were endowed with a facet of divinity. That is what gives us knowledge of our immortality.

You should live until you die.

No one dies alone.

Everyone is loved beyond comprehension.

Everyone is blessed and guided.

It is very important that you do only what you love to do. You may be poor, you may go hungry, you may live in a shabby place, but you will totally live. And at the end of your days, you will bless your life because you have done what you came here to do.

The hardest lesson to learn is unconditional love.

Dying is nothing to fear. It can be the most wonderful experience of your life. It all depends on how you have lived.

Death is but a transition from this life to another existence where there is no more pain and anguish.

Everything is bearable when there is love.

My wish is that you try to give more people more love.

The only thing that lives forever is love.